SURVIVING BABY LOSS WHILE BATTLING INFERTILITY

Inspired by a Real Story

KIALI J. GARRETT

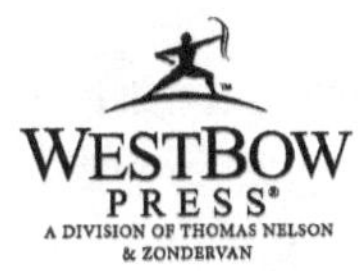

WESTBOW PRESS®
A DIVISION OF THOMAS NELSON
& ZONDERVAN

WestBow Press books may be ordered through booksellers or by contacting:

WestBow Press
A Division of Thomas Nelson & Zondervan
1663 Liberty Drive
Bloomington, IN 47403
www.westbowpress.com
844-714-3454

ISBN: 978-1-6642-4412-2 (sc)
ISBN: 978-1-6642-4411-5 (hc)
ISBN: 978-1-6642-4413-9 (e)

Library of Congress Control Number: 2021918193

Print information available on the last page.

WestBow Press rev. date: 10/20/2021

DEDICATION

This book is dedicated to my angel baby boy, who although never had the opportunity to open his eyes and see life beyond my womb, has taught me so many lessons that I will forever cherish. Gone but not forgotten, forever in our hearts. To God be the Glory!

ACKNOWLEDGEMENTS

Praises, honor and thanks to the almighty God for seeing me through the darkest moments of my life and for filling me with wisdom, knowledge, and strength to be able to share my unique circumstances with the world.

Profound gratitude to you my amazing husband Felix, for your unconditional love, unwavering support, and endless prayers. You've shown me that a good companion shortens the longest road ever traveled. Thank you for standing by me, for encouraging me, for giving me an extra push whenever I need it and above all, thank you for being you. You are a super star!

A deep-rooted sense of gratitude and indebtedness to my family for standing by me during this challenging, yet enriching period of my life. You are my oasis……. that safe place that I always return to in order to recuperate and to reorient my steps. I thank God for blessing me with you all.

My dear friends, you guys are remarkable and I'm so grateful to have you in my life. Thank you for all the love, support, compassion and understanding that you provided during this journey. I appreciate you more than you can ever imagine.

To all the lovely ladies I met during my fertility journey, you are amazing. Your unique circumstances made me understand how important this topic is and solidified the fact that my story is valid and worth sharing.

A massive thank you to the editorial team at WestBow Press for helping me bring this project to life. Your professionalism, attention to detail and commitment are a force to be reckoned with and I am grateful that our paths crossed.

WHAT THIS BOOK IS ABOUT

A real story inspired by some adversities that I have encountered in my life and how I managed to triumph over them to get to where I am today.

MOTIVATION

Taking into consideration the joy, unexpected pain, and emotional trauma I have experienced, I've always believed that I have important things to say—things that women need to hear, things that men need to hear, things that young adults need to hear, and things that the world at large needs to hear. Unfortunately, my story is wrapped around stigmatized topics that are uncomfortable to talk about and still considered taboos in the world we live in today.

These, unfortunately, are topics that most people shy away from having conversations about. They are shrouded in mystery and, sadly, shame. We shouldn't feel ashamed or be made to feel ashamed about things we didn't bestow on ourselves or things we have absolutely no control over whatsoever. We should be able to express ourselves without being labeled—at least one would think so, but it's hardly ever the case because we live in constant fear and never truly express ourselves once we believe our narrative is knotted to a stigmatized subject.

Fearful of the fact that I will be named and shamed if I open up about my struggles, I decided to hide behind my computer and seek support from online communities made up of incredible people with similar struggles. Like almost every other member of these online communities, my exchanges were anonymous. In as much as these communities provided a safe place for me and other members to vent freely without any fear, guilt, or embarrassment, I still felt like a prisoner. I wasn't completely free. I wasn't able to put my name and face to my own struggles, and I wasn't the only one. Approximately 98 percent of those using these platforms didn't either. They used fake names and random pictures on their profiles.

I wanted to be able to talk about my struggles and feelings to friends and family, but I couldn't, and this was frustrating, detrimental, and devastating on all levels. Nothing about it felt right to me. I didn't want to live the rest of my life feeling this way. I had to crunch this hideous, gruesome monster of a taboo, but what I didn't know was how to go about it. *How do I break this stigma and come forward with my struggles?* That was the ultimate question I kept asking myself. After long and deep thoughts, I finally came to the realization that a book would be the best way to share my story, as I could take my time to carefully generate and craft the content that would bring it out in as much detail as possible.

In the process of trying to figure out the best way to let the cat out of the bag, I stumbled on Bryony Gordon's *Mad World* podcast of April 2017 titled, "Why It's Totally Normal to Feel Weird." (*Bryony Gordon's Mad World: Prince Harry on Apple Podcasts.*)

Dealing with a roller coaster of emotions and feeling weird, I could obviously use a good laugh and take some notes from something with such a captivating topic. I hit the pause button and made myself a good hot cup of green tea to sip on while taking a listen to what I thought would be some incredibly brilliant comedy.

To my greatest astonishment, Bryony's first guest was Prince Harry. My curiosity was aroused even more, and I couldn't wait to hear what the prince had to say about "why it's totally normal to feel weird." The chitchat I had set out to enjoy and get a good laugh from turned out to be the absolute unexpected—a rare, extraordinary, and very candid interview, one in which Harry defied the British royal tradition by opening up about years of pain as he struggled to manage his life and mental health issues.

I'm not sure Bryony expected the prince to be that candid. In the podcast interview, Harry went personal and inconceivably deep. He disclosed that the loss of his mother was directly linked to the difficulties he experienced in his life and that he actually had to seek professional help to come to terms with it. Given the fact that the royal family is well known for upholding a long-standing motto, "Never explain, never complain," I was completely blown away by the words the prince was uttering.

Verbatim, the prince said, "I can safely say that losing my mom at the age of twelve, and therefore shutting down all my emotions for the last twenty years, has had a quite serious effect on not only my personal life but my work as well." Striking, isn't it? Although it took the prince two long decades to come to terms with the underlying cause of his suffering and struggles, he acknowledged that his inward feelings had been on display the entire time through his outward behavior, but sadly enough, Harry couldn't put his finger on it. "I just didn't know what was wrong with me," he said.

You probably (*maybe not*) remember the days when the prince was in his twenties and creating a buzz. He regularly made headlines on the news for not-so-very-pleasant things, most especially because he comes from the royal family. Had he been born into a regular middle-class family, for example, there is a high possibility that no one would've bothered about who he was, what he did, or what he didn't do. He did things that are not alien to most young adults, but coming from the royal family shifts gears to be held to higher standards.

It was very common for the prince to be on the news for getting wild at drunken parties, smoking pot, having well-oiled evenings with a series of beautiful young women in revealing outfits, and even attending a costume ball in a Nazi uniform. Now, that's more than enough to give the queen a heart attack, but thank goodness, she survived this trying period.

Harry also disclosed that things started to change for him when he was finally able to evoke the loss of his mother and the inner anger with specialized therapists where he opened up about the emotions he had kept bottled up for decades. I don't know about you, but this directly hit home for me. I had emotions bottled up that I couldn't express because of the stigma they carried. Listening to this podcast and learning that this ostrich policy could eventually lead to severe psychological effects got my wheels turning and my imagination running wild as I tried to fathom the depth of the prince's candid acknowledgments.

If such a high-profile public figure as Prince Harry can defy the tradition of one of the most respected families in the world in order to come forward with his struggles, I have no reason to remain in the closet. Unlike the prince, I am a common citizen with no long-lasting tradition or motto to uphold and no image to protect. What then is my excuse for not being able to divulge? The taboo to speak up about stigmatized topics? Not anymore. From then onward, I promised myself that prejudice and fear would no longer stand in my way. If anything, I would transform my pain into a meaningful life experience that people in similar situations could benefit from.

In my opinion, Prince Harry's candid admission is directly from the heart for a cause. It emerged as he campaigned for the Heads Together mental health charity championed by himself and his brother and sister-in-law, Prince William and Kate (the duke and duchess of Cambridge), working to eradicate the stigma around mental health problems. Taking the prince's past personal scuffles with mental health into consideration, he decided to put his name and face to the stigma surrounding this issue. He understands how important this issue is because he has experienced it firsthand. He knows how it feels to not be able to talk about how you truly feel.

He articulates that he is so passionate about this cause because there are many people struggling with the stigma who are afraid to admit it for fear of prejudice and judgment. His goal is to change the national conversation on mental well-being so that people can feel free to talk about their feelings without fear.

I'm pretty sure that Harry wasn't thinking about me when he gave that interview. Like Helen Adams Keller rightly put it, "When we do the best we can, we never know what miracle is wrought in our life or in the life of another." Thank you, Prince Harry, for taking stock of your struggles and opening up to the world, assuring people like me and many others that we are not the only ones dealing with difficult, stigmatized situations. Many other strong, successful, high-profile public figures also suffer their own stigmatized difficulties, but the difference is that just a few people like you openly talk about it. Your move is a constant reminder to me that I am not alone.

Today I know not to keep a stiff upper lip at the expense of my well-being. I know not to bend my head anymore because of my struggles. I know to hold my head up high and look the world straight in the eye because of what you did.

CONTENTS

PHASE 1

Unexpected Loss and Its Aftermath

(Inspired by My Unique Experience)

CHAPTER 1

The Wake-Up Call

It wasn't a regular private practice that Christina was accustomed to, one where the doctor will proudly hang a sign outside the practice with his or her name on it followed by *MD*. Such doctors have the autonomy to decide what hours they work, which insurance to accept, which patients to see, and how much to charge for their services. Such American doctors have their own practices, which they are able to operate as they choose. Things are a little different in some other parts of the world. In the United Arab Emirates, where Christina lives, there's a lot to adjust to, including the health care system.

In essence, UAE doctors are hospital employees with very attractive fixed salaries, which spaces them out from some of the unpredictable changes in health care, especially in North America. In most cases, this can be a relief, especially for a doctor who no longer has to fear nearby competing practices or insurance companies that may be cutting physician reimbursements. That said, Christina no longer has to drive to a doctor's office like she did in the United States; she now drives to an actual hospital building whenever she has to visit a doctor.

It has been a routine for a couple of months now. Once every two weeks, Christina drives to Shamsa Hospital for her doctor's visit. Whenever she pulls up to the front entrance of the hospital, she is greeted by professional-looking and smiling valets who are ready to offer their services. They are always dressed in tailored chocolate-brown pants and crisp,- white short-sleeved shirts with brown shoulder pads and yellow straps on them. One could easily mistake them for security guards except that they all wear name tags with *Shamsa Valet Services* boldly engraved on them. In addition, these guys are always happy. You would think they have the best jobs in the world.

Once the vehicle is no longer in motion, one of the valets will walk close to the car and carefully place a ticket on the windshield, securing it with the windshield wiper. He will then proceed to the driver and give her another ticket, reminding her to get a stamp from the doctor's office after her visit in order to not be charged for valet services. Christina will thank them and step out of the car, handing the keys over to the valet.

She will then walk through the automatic door, head straight to the elevator, hit the up arrow, and wait for the elevator to come down. Sometimes she will be waiting with a lot of people, and sometimes not. Regardless, there are six very large elevators, each with a 4,500-kilogram (9,900-pound) capacity, serving the twenty-six-floor building, so vertical travel from one floor to the other is fairly easy.

As Christina and other patients stand in line, almost everyone lifts up their heads from time to time to check how close the elevator is to the ground floor. After a very short wait, beeping signals the elevator has arrived. Everyone is ready to hop on and head to their floors of interest, but for courtesy, they have to wait for people to exit first. Once they all exit, Christina hops on and presses the button for the second floor.

The second floor has a couple of other clinics, but Christina is bound for the gynecology section where her doctor is based. She arrives at the clinic, signs in with the receptionist, and takes a seat as she waits for her turn. A few minutes later, she hears her name being said in a sentence: "Madame Christina Jonas assessment. Madame Christina Jonas assessment."

Christina stands up and looks around, holding her handbag in one hand and her mobile phone in the other. As she looks around, she locks eyes with a brown-skinned, medium-height, dark-haired, middle-aged lady in pink scrubs standing by a half-open door with a sign at the top that reads: "Assessment." She looks like someone of Filipino decent but is definitely Asian.

The lady smiles at her, and Christina smiles back.

She asks, "Are you Madame Christina?"

Christina replies reluctantly in bewilderment, "Yes, I am."

Being addressed as *madame* is not something she fancies or is accustomed to. However, it is customary in this region to address women as *madame* and men as *sir*. To the locals, it displays a great deal of respect, which they desire so much that they become exasperated when addressed directly by name. On the contrary, Christina doesn't like being called *madame*. But as the saying goes, "When in Rome, do as the Romans do." She has no choice other than to adapt and roll with the punches.

The lady asks Christina to come in for an assessment. The assessment is a quick process that lasts approximately five minutes. Blood pressure, oxygen level, weight, and height are taken and recorded, and a few questions are asked about the reason for the visit. Christina is then asked to go back to the waiting area until she is called in to see the doctor.

And as usual, the wait turns out to be a long one.

Generally speaking, she prefers morning appointments because they usually have fewer people with shorter wait times. Anyone who has been to a doctor's office knows about the painfully long waits. For example, you may have a 10:00 a.m. appointment and sign in by 9:45 a.m., thinking you'll be called in right around ten. Sadly, that's hardly ever the case. The truth is there may be a handful of people in the waiting area with appointments within the same time slot—such a classic example of chronic overscheduling.

One of my doctors, in an effort to explain why we often experience long wait times at doctors' offices, told me that doctors generally come out of school with the same amount of debt as their friends who have entered more lucrative specialties. The only way to make up for some of the difference and pay back their loans is to see more patients; hence, patients are scheduled closer together. She further explained that this normally doesn't cause problems with the schedule or increase wait times significantly, but life happens.

If the doctor is one with hospital privileges and goes to deliveries, emergencies will happen. That doctor will have to prioritize each situation and respond with immediate effect. She said, "Getting called to a C-section, for example, can ruin the schedule for a busy practice." Whatever the reason for the long waits may be, the fact remains that it has huge ramifications on the waiting patients' experience regarding that visit and the practice in general.

Some thirty-five minutes later, Christina hears her name again.

"Madame Christina Jonas." The sound seems to have emerged from her left, so she immediately turns her head and looks in that direction. She finds a slightly open door with a little smiling lady's head and neck extending out of the door. The rest of her body can barely be seen. She is also in pink scrubs and has long, silky black hair pulled back in a neat ponytail. Still smiling, she says, "Madame Christina?"

Christina nods her head, walks to the door, and is ushered into the room by the nurse.

It's a massive room, approximately 350 square feet with wall-to-wall windows and a really nice setup for a doctor's office. Simply put, this office is fancy. The doctor is sitting behind a beautiful, gigantic desk with two large monitors. She stands up and says, "It's always a pleasure to see you *habibti* (meaning *sweetheart* in Arabic). How are you doing today?"

"Very well, Doctor. How about yourself? How are you doing?"

"I'm fine. Have a seat, habibti."

They proceed to chat about random stuff for about a minute, laughing in between, before going to the reason for the visit: ultrasound monitoring. Christina finds her to be such a pleasant and warm doctor—one she can feel comfortable with, which is a fundamental factor as she goes through this phase.

Christina had been put on oral ovulation-inducing medications approximately two weeks ago and is now back for a follow-up. During this visit, the doctor conducts an ultrasound to check the development of her ovarian follicles. She finds two visible, dominant, mature follicles measuring twenty-two millimeters and twenty-four millimeters. She likes what she is seeing and is excited for Christina.

"We have a very good shot this cycle," says the doctor. "I will write you a prescription for an HCG [human chorionic gonadotropic] injection to initiate the release of the eggs and the development of the corpus luteum, which will help your body produce progesterone."

Christina replies, "Thank you, Doctor." Candidly, she doesn't quite understand all the parlance the doctor has just spilled, but she understands enough to grasp the general concept, and that's acceptable.

Upon finishing with the ultrasound, the doctor walks back to her seat while Christina gets dressed and ultimately joins her at her desk. The doctor then scribbles a prescription on a piece of letterhead and hands it to

Christina, saying, "Go down to the pharmacy, buy this injection, and take it to the ninth floor, where the nurse will administer it for you."

Christina takes a quick glance at the prescription. She can barely read what the doctor has written but doesn't bother to ask. *All doctors write like that anyway. I'm pretty sure the pharmacists can read it,* she thinks to herself.

The doctor adds, "Ovulation usually occurs approximately twenty-four to thirty-six hours after the HCG injection is administered. To maximize your chances, intercourse is mandatory for you today, tomorrow, and the day after." At this point, the doctor stretches both hands out to Christina, holds her hands tightly, and says as she looks her straight in the eyes, "You will be pregnant this month *inshallah* [meaning *God willing* in Arabic]. I will be praying for you, habibti."

"Thank you so much, Doctor." Christina replies. She then rushes to the pharmacy, purchases her injection, and heads to the ninth floor as instructed.

As she is sitting in a small room on the ninth floor waiting for the nurse to come administer the trigger shot, she becomes carried away in thought. She envisions herself getting a positive pregnancy test in two weeks, her belly growing as weeks and months pass by, and eventually having a baby nine months down the road, and the rest is a phantasmagoria. She is elated. "I can't believe it's finally happening," she says to herself.

Suddenly, the door opened, and Christina skips with terror as her right hand speedily races for her chest in an effort to ease the shock waves that just ran through her heart and body.

"Are you okay?" The nurse asks.

"Yeah … yeah. You scared me a little, bit but I'm okay. I just got lost in some deep thoughts, but I'm fine."

"Oh! Sorry about that. My name is Jasmine. I'm the nurse, and I'm here to administer your injection," she explains.

"I know," replies Christina.

The nurse smiles as she pulls out the injection from the ice-filled plastic bag. One glance at the package, and the nurse immediately knows what it is for. She lifts her head and turns to Christina with a question. "How long have you been trying?"

Mind you, Christina did not like being asked this question. Each time someone asked her, it brought back sad memories of the unfortunate placental abruption she suffered that led to the loss of her beautiful baby boy. As a result, she ponders things such as why it occurred, why isn't her baby here, and why she needs help getting pregnant? Those thoughts linger for a while.

Although her mood has been rendered dismal by the question, she manages to fake a smile that appears very genuine and replies, "A few months now."

The nurse smiles at her and says, "*Inshallah* [God willing] this injection will help you this month."

"Thank you," Christina replies.

The nurse administers the injection, and Christina thanks her and exits the room.

On her way home, Christina starts revisiting the events that led to this struggle bus she now finds herself on. In retrospect, her first pregnancy wasn't planned. She got pregnant during her first month of marriage, but she experienced a complete placental abruption on August 4, 2014, in the thirty-seventh week of her pregnancy, and sadly, her baby didn't make it. Due to the severity of the abruption, doctors advised that it was best to wait for at least twelve to eighteen months before trying for another baby, as it was very important for her body to heal.

Although Christina and Tim respect the doctor's recommendation, it certainly isn't a walk in the park. It is a long, cold, and miserable wait filled with shock, grief, frustration, guilt, depression, a sense of failure, confusion, and even vulnerability. No, waiting is not the problem here, maintaining sanity while waiting is the problem. What is she even supposed to do during this waiting period? What is the right thing to do while waiting, if there is any such thing as the right thing? How can you move forward with such a heavy heart? How can she comport herself in the process when she can't take her mind off the loss? It is such a horrific situation to be in.

Eventually, eighteen months come and pass, and Christina goes to her doctor for the long-awaited follow-up appointment regarding her healing process. Amazingly, she has healed properly. In the doctor's own words, "Everything looks good to me. You've healed very nicely. I think you can start trying again whenever you feel like it."

Christina is ecstatic by the sound of these words. She calls her husband as soon as she sets foot out of the doctor's office with the news, and he is delighted too. They'd been looking forward to this day, praying and hoping for an all-clear report, and now they have it.

CHAPTER 2

Before the Abruption

Life before the abruption is uneventful for Christina and Tim. In as much as they love planning for the future, there is one thing that is not in their plan: conceive a baby and end up losing the baby to a complete placental abruption at thirty-eight weeks. As a matter of fact, no matter how meticulous of a planner one can be, no one factors in such items in their plans. You don't make a plan for an unexpected loss. It just happens to you.

Thrilled at the realization that they are expecting a baby, they can hardly wait to make it to three months in order to share the news with their family and friends. Quite frankly, the three-month period isn't one where they are discussing fears of anything happening to the pregnancy. It is one filled with incredible joy, anticipation, and eagerness to let their beautiful secret out.

At three months along, they share the news with their loved ones, and everyone is elated and can't wait to welcome baby. There is not a single moment when they envision something negative will snatch their baby from them within the twinkle of an eye. They are excited and busy planning for their baby's arrival, brainstorming names, coming up with ideas about what the nursery will look like, and envisioning their lives with a precious little one.

While they are not oblivious about mishaps that could occur in a pregnancy, they aren't fully informed about them either. They've heard a thing or two about early loses (miscarriages), especially within the first three months of conception, but not very much about loses after the three-month mark. All along, they've been surrounded by couples who've welcomed babies into their families with no real issues to be concerned about, and they believe that life is as such. You get pregnant, make it to three months, announce your pregnancy, and welcome a beautiful baby six months later. That's exactly what Christina and Tim are focused on while living a healthy lifestyle and keeping doctor's appointments.

As soon as Christina finds out she is pregnant, she schedules her first appointment with the doctor who confirms her pregnancy, reviews her symptoms (barely any are present), takes her medical history, and collects urine and blood samples.

The urine samples are collected to check for the presence of any bacteria, high sugar levels, and high protein levels. If the sugar levels are high, it could be a sign of diabetes, and if protein levels are high, it could be a sign of preeclampsia, which is a type of high blood pressure that occurs during pregnancy. The blood samples are collected to check for things such as blood cell counts, blood type, anemia (low iron levels), and infectious diseases, such as HIV, hepatitis, and syphilis.

Apart from urine and blood samples and taking into consideration Christina's background, the doctor also conducts a pelvic exam to check the size and shape of her uterus, and everything looks good to her. She also does a pap smear to screen for cervical cancer and an ultrasound to view the baby's position and to measure his or her growth. This is Christina's favorite part of the visit, as it gives her an opportunity to spot an image of her baby on a video screen for the first time. She is enraptured. As a matter of fact, she remembers telling the doctor, "I can watch this movie forever and not get bored or tired because it's so beautiful."

A few days later, all test results are in, and everything looks good. Her numbers are terrific, and her doctor is happy. There are no bacteria detected in Christina's urine; her sugar levels are within a perfect range, which eliminates any signs of diabetes; and there are no signs of preeclampsia, infectious diseases, or cervical cancer. She has an all-clear report.

Christina continues her prenatal care and keeps visiting her doctor every four weeks with the above-mentioned tests being repeated periodically, always with immaculate results as her pregnancy progresses. During these visits, some things are standard; her weight is taken, her blood pressure is checked, her urine is collected and examined, the baby's heartbeat is listened to, and the uterus is measured to monitor baby's growth.

During months seven and eight, doctor's visits become more frequent, and Christina now goes in every other week. At month nine, however, the visits become even more frequent, and she is now seen on a weekly basis. Even at this advanced stage of Christina's pregnancy, everything continues to be perfect, without a single red flag to signal that things were about to springboard downhill in just a week.

By this time, preparations are almost done. The crib has been picked out, and the nursery has been beautifully decorated. Baby's closet is ready with the cutest little outfits that mommy, daddy, grandpa, grandma, uncles, aunties, friends, colleagues of Christina and Tim, and well-wishers in general have purchased. There are even some crocheted outfits that have been carefully handcrafted by Grandma with a whole lot of love and care. Baby's stroller, car seat, and diaper bag are about to be shipped out from California to Baltimore where baby will be born.

What was Christina's prenatal care routine like?

The norm is that you are more likely to have a healthy birth if you maintain a healthy pregnancy, right? There is even a fancy term for it: prenatal care. Christina understands the importance of maintaining a healthy pregnancy and does everything expected and more to take care of herself and her unborn baby during this incredibly exhilarating period of her life. Join me as I take a deeper dive into her prenatal routine.

What is in her pill box?

Folic acid is the number one pill in Christina's pill box, and she takes it religiously. As you may already know, health professionals recommend that pregnant women should be taking at least 400 micrograms (mcg) of folic acid every day during the entire pregnancy to help prevent problems with baby's brain and spine.

What is her diet like?

Christina is normally a healthy eater; however, during her pregnancy, her focus is not only on eating healthy but also on making sure she is eating a balanced diet in order to provide her body the nutrients it needs to function properly and maintain a healthy pregnancy. Most of her calorie intake comes from fresh fruit and vegetables (especially dark, leafy greens), whole grains, legumes, dairy, nuts, and lean protein.

She avoids highly processed foods, refined grains, added sugar and salt, processed meats, foods high in mercury, alcohol, caffeine, and trans fats. Simply put, she avoids empty-calorie foods.

Adopting the above eating habits gives her confidence that she is nourishing her body with essential vitamins, minerals, antioxidants, carbohydrates (including starches and fiber), protein, and healthy fats that are crucial to eating a balanced diet. These changes also give her peace of mind that she is doing the best thing for herself and her baby during this exciting period of her life.

How about exercise?

It is no secret to Christina that exercise promotes a healthy lifestyle and can help ease discomfort. She's even heard that exercising while pregnant makes labor and delivery easier, but she can't speak much about this because she didn't go into labor. You get the vibe? Let's stick with what we can back with our own unique experiences.

With Christina being an active individual prior to getting pregnant coupled with the fact that she has no issues with this pregnancy, her doctor determines that it is safe for her to continue exercising. That said, she tries her best to get in at least thirty minutes of exercise every day (except for a few where she falls off the wagon), making sure she hydrates herself very well in the process and that she listens to her body in case she develops any discomfort from being active. Thankfully, she has nothing to report.

Has she gained weight?

Weight gain during pregnancy is different for every pregnant woman. The general recommendation is that pregnant women should gain anywhere between twenty-five to thirty pounds, more if the woman is underweight and less if the woman is overweight. This, however, is often left to each individual's doctor's discretion because they know what's best for their patients. Taking Christina's prepregnancy weight into consideration, she falls within the acceptable weight gain range, which is fantastic.

How about work?

Although pregnancy is not an illness and shouldn't be viewed as one, it is important to understand that a woman's overall health plays a role in how late in her pregnancy she can continue to work without putting herself or her unborn baby at risk. The type of job the woman has and the environment she works in all play a role. For example, women with active jobs may not be able to work as long as women with less active jobs. Jobs that involve radiation, lead, and other harmful materials such as copper and mercury are not safe to continue to perform while pregnant, as they can be harmful to the baby.

Christina is determined to be in overall great health, and she has a nine-to-five desk job in an environment free of toxins. She works for the first five months of her pregnancy and then quits her job in order to move up north to be with her family where she will give birth to her baby.

What symptoms does she experience?

It's infrequent to talk to a pregnant woman who isn't experiencing a symptom or two or even several; sometimes, the symptoms are too many to count. The majority of these symptoms surface within the first trimester when a woman's body is struggling to adjust to raging hormones. Some women even begin to experience symptoms before they miss a period. This is usually great news for those who are actively trying to conceive and maybe not great news for those who either do not want any more babies, do not want babies at all, or do not want babies that particular time in their lives.

There are a whole lot of symptoms that come with pregnancy with obvious ones being a missed period, tender breasts, nausea with or without vomiting, fatigue, and increased urination. Other symptoms such as cramping, food aversions, bloating, constipation, moodiness, light spotting, and nasal congestion, although considered less obvious in general terms, can sometimes be unbearable for some expectant mothers. Every woman is different, and every pregnancy, even for the same woman, is different.

When asked about symptoms and side effects of pregnancy, Christina says she considers herself one of the lucky few because although she did experience some discomfort, it wasn't extraordinary compared to what others go through during pregnancy. She only remembers having a few of the above-mentioned symptoms as she highlights in the following paragraphs.

Increased Urination

I often joke that my kidneys worked overtime on purpose when I was pregnant. They made sure to stay busy just so they could process extra fluid to deposit into my bladder. It felt like my bladder was just never empty no matter how many times I went to the bathroom. I was always on some sort of a bathroom break. I couldn't walk around the mall without looking for a bathroom sign, and I hardly stopped to pump gas without swinging by the restroom. I sort of lived in bathrooms during my pregnancy. It was so annoying that drinking water or ingesting liquids in general began feeling a like a chore. It took a lot of discipline to keep myself hydrated.

Food Aversions and Cravings

I became more sensitive to certain odors, and my sense of taste changed. Certain foods I used to enjoy just didn't smell or taste good to me anymore. I could not stand greasy food, meat, or orange juice.

On the flip side, while I never really had an overpowering longing for any food in particular during the majority of my pregnancy, I found myself beginning to relish okra, and this is something I have never liked. My taste buds definitely went haywire. Growing up, whenever okra was on the menu, mom will prepare a different meal for me.

Toward the end of my third trimester, I started having an overpowering longing for croissants. There were times when I would do some legendary middle-of-the-night runs to the kitchen for croissants. My Sweet Mother made sure we never ran out of them. Whenever she went grocery shopping, she would come home with a jumbo box from the store. Isn't she just the sweetest?!

Apart from food aversions, I also remember how my favorite scent all of a sudden started to smell caustic at one point. It got so bad that I stopped wearing perfume until my pregnancy came to an end.

Bloating

Early on in my pregnancy I felt very bloated—sort of how you might feel at the start of your menstrual period. If you have ever experienced this feeling, before you know it's not pretty. Thank goodness this symptom/side effect was occasional and only lasted a few months. I wonder what I would have done if it persisted.

Constipation

I wrestled with constipation the entire time. I would eat fiber-rich foods and drink a lot of water and other liquids and still wound up constipated. Metamucil was doing the job, but then it began tasting awful I would feel sick to my stomach just looking at that orange container.

I cannot count how many times I was tempted to pop some Dulcolax pills in my mouth just to get some relief. I even contemplated a tea made especially for dieters that was packaged in a green box picturing a skinny woman striking a sophisticated yoga pose on a teacup. I thought this tea was a great idea because it read "no caffeine." I am glad this urge was purged at the contemplative phase. If I had gone further and taken that tea and later suffered the abruption, I would have blamed things on the tea and carried that load forever.

Speaking to my doctor about all these discomforts, I was advised that hormones were expected to soar during pregnancy, so everything was chalked up to hormonal changes. What I was experiencing were classic pregnancy symptoms and side effects that would eventually fade away after I gave birth, and sure enough, they did fade away.

A Little Question and Answer Session with Christina

When you are pregnant, there are various things that you should avoid in order to maintain a healthy pregnancy. Let us take a look at some of these dangerous habits.

Smoking, for example, increases a pregnant women's risk of having a miscarriage, preterm labor, low birth weight, and other health problems.

Cocaine, marijuana, heroin, and other drugs equally raise the risk of a miscarriage, preterm labor, and birth defects. It is not uncommon for women who continue to use drugs while pregnant to give birth to babies with an addiction to the drugs they have been abusing while pregnant. Such a condition is called neonatal abstinence syndrome and is very likely to cause severe health problems for the baby.

Consuming alcohol while pregnant is one of the major causes of preventable birth defects up to and including fetal alcohol disorder.

Based on that information, Christina participated in a little Q&A session to give us a better understanding of her lifestyle choices.

Question: Do you smoke?

Answer: No, I have never smoked in my life.

Question: Do you use drugs?

Answer: No, I do not, and I have never used drugs.

Question: Do you drink alcohol?

Answer: Socially, not heavily, and very rarely too.

The Last Stretch

At month seven, doctor's visits become more frequent. Christina goes in every other week, which continues through month eight. At month nine, however, the visits become even more frequent, and she is now seen on a weekly basis. Even at this advanced stage of Christina's pregnancy, everything continues to be perfect with not a single red flag to signal that things were about to springboard downhill in just a week.

By this time, as you would rightly imagine, preparations are almost done. The crib has been picked out, and the nursery has been beautifully decorated. Baby's closet is ready with the cutest little outfits that mommy, daddy, grandpa, grandma, siblings, uncles, aunties, friends, colleagues, and well-wishers in general have purchased. There are even some crocheted outfits that have been carefully handcrafted by Grandma with a whole lot of love and care. Baby's stroller, car seat, and diaper bag are about to be shipped out from California to Baltimore.

Preparations and anticipation continue mounting until August 4, 2014, when things take a painful sharp turn downhill—one that will change Christina's life forever.

CHAPTER 3

The Dreaded Placental Abruption

The single most important resource for a woman's fetus is her placenta. It provides protection and nourishment to her developing fetus. It is basically the baby's lifeline, and any disruption to that lifeline could have negative implications, ranging from developmental delays or a miscarriage to, worst-case scenario, an abruption. An abruption can either be partial or full. A partial abruption occurs when the placenta detaches itself from the uterine lining in part, and a complete abruption occurs when the placenta detaches itself from the uterine lining in full. Either situation is one of the most frightening pregnancy complications that a pregnant woman can encounter. This condition usually occurs in the third trimester, but it could occur at any time after the twentieth week of pregnancy. Only about 1 percent of all pregnant women are likely to experience a placental abruption, and most can be successfully treated depending on the kind of separation the woman suffers.

What Causes Placental Abruption?

Although the causes of placental abruption are not commonly known, pregnant women in general are at a risk for this condition if they smoke, use cocaine during pregnancy, have preeclampsia (hypertension), are older than thirty-five, are pregnant with multiples, have had a previous placental abruption, have some abnormalities in the uterus, or have experienced trauma to the abdomen during the pregnancy.

Monday, August 4, 2014, is a day Christina and Tim will never forget. It is the day their world came crashing down abruptly and unexpectedly. Tim has traveled for work and has been gone for a week now. Christina wakes up strong and healthy as usual. Baby is kicking strong and healthy in Christina's womb as well. She receives her regular morning call from Tim and jump-starts her day. She is thirty-seven weeks and five days far along and has her weekly prenatal visit today.

Excited as ever, she drives to her doctor's appointment. All checks are done, and mother and baby are determined to be doing great. The doctor tells Christina that she is 2 centimeters dilated, and the possibility of her baby coming early is very high. She instructs Christina to go straight to the labor and delivery unit should labor kick in before her due date. She adds that because Christina has been seeing a different doctor before moving to Baltimore, she will order a repeat glucose test for her. Christina goes to the lab located on the first floor of the same building to get the test done.

While at the lab, the lab technician informs her that the test will take one hour to complete. She proceeds to take a blood sample to measure Christina's baseline glucose level. Immediately after that, she gives her a sugary solution called Glucola and instructs her to drink all of it within the next five minutes. Christina is accustomed to this procedure, as she has taken the test before. Upon finishing the drink, the lab technician says, "Take a seat in the waiting area, and I will call you in after sixty minutes to take another blood sample."

"Okay," replies Christina.

Approximately fifteen minutes into the wait, Christina starts feeling uncomfortable. Her stomach doesn't feel right, and she feels like vomiting. She tries to suppress the feeling, but it is persistent. This is such a strange feeling. She is nearly thirty-eight weeks along and hasn't experienced any nausea of any kind thus far—not even the morning sickness. Her pregnancy has been perfect all along. She knows her body and definitely believes something is wrong.

She attempts to walk up to notify the lab technician who stops her from a distance in an angry tone and says, "Ma'am, I told you I will call you in after sixty minutes."

"I feel like throwing up," replies Christina.

"If you throw up, you will have to repeat the test, and I really don't have the time to repeat your test because I have to take my lunch break. Just sit down and wait until the sixty-minute period is over," says the technician with a stinky attitude.

Christina can feel the discomfort escalating. She rushes into the bathroom and tries to throw up, but nothing comes out. She lingers around for a while in the bathroom to no avail. Frustrated, she runs up to the doctor's office to give a report on how she feels. Unfortunately, the doctor has stepped out to respond to an emergency in the hospital. The nurses tell her it will calm down and that she should go back to the lab and complete the test.

At the sixtieth minute, the lab technician calls her in, draws some blood, and discharges her to go home. Christina sluggishly walks to her car. The feeling continues to get worse, and she can feel her energy level plummeting. She tries to drive herself home but physically can't, as she feels her body getting weaker and weaker. She feels a desperate need to throw up, but nothing happens. There is mounting pressure from the nausea, and she feels helpless. She calls her mother and tells her how she feels. Sweet Mother advises her not to drive, fetches her car keys, and immediately gets on the road to go get her.

Approximately fifteen minutes later, she pulls up in the parking lot. Christina is sort of feeling better by now. The nausea is subsiding, and she feels her nerves gradually calming down. She is convinced it was the Glucola that didn't agree with her system. Her mom assists her out of the car and into the passenger seat of her own car, and they enjoy a smooth ride home.

As they walk into the house hand in hand, Christina's mom turns to her and asks, "Sunroom?"

Christina nods her head in approval, smiling. Her mom then leads her to the sunroom and onto the couch. This is Christina's favorite room in the house, and Sweet Mother knows that. It is decorated with Christina's favorite decor colors: olive green and ivory. She loves to lie down on the olive green four-seater couch, which, in her opinion, is strategically placed in the room. It gives her a perfect view of the street, the backyard, and the television. She feels very relaxed whenever she sits on this couch.

Sweet Mother has even gone the extra mile to make the room more inviting and comfortable for Christina and her big belly. As she lies on the couch, caressing her huge belly, Sweet Mother rushes upstairs and comes back down with more pillows and a nice cover just to make sure Christina is as comfortable as can be. She always thinks of those little but very imperative things that most people will hardly think of.

As soon as Sweet Mother finishes propping Christina with the pillows, Christina's phone rings. It's Tim calling to check on how the appointment went. He didn't like missing any appointments, but sometimes life happens, and we have to take it a day at a time. Christina doesn't sound good on the phone. He can sense it even before she tells him.

"What's the matter, honey?" asks Tim.

"I'm not feeling too good today. Nausea is getting the better of me. I feel like I want to throw up, but it just doesn't happen," replies Christina. She continues by narrating the lab incident to Tim.

"Don't worry about anything. Just focus on feeling better. You are approximately two weeks away from having the baby, so hang in there please. It will be over soon, honey," says Tim. They continue to chat for a little bit before getting off the phone.

Still lying down, Christina feels some discomfort in her stomach. She also feels hard-pressed. She gets up and slowly makes her way to the bathroom to relieve herself. While in the bathroom, she feels a sharp, excruciating pain in her stomach that makes her scream at the top of her voice. Sweet Mother runs to the bathroom and finds Christina sitting on the commode with tears running down her cheeks.

"Please, Sweet Mother. Come closer and help me up. I'm finding it challenging to stand up on my own," cries Christina.

Her Sweet Mother helps her up, assists her out to the living room, and lays her down on the closest couch.

"I'm taking you to the hospital right away. The baby might be coming early. Give me a minute to grab my purse, and let's go," says Sweet Mother. As she runs for her purse, Christina can feel the pain level increasing at the speed of light. It feels like her body is on pins, needles, and fire all at the same time. Everything is happening so fast.

"Call the ambulance instead, Sweet Mother. Please! Call the ambulance. I feel like someone is piercing needles all over my body," screams Christina.

"Okay, babe, let me do that right away," replies Sweet Mother as she scuffles with the phone in an effort to dial 911. In less than five minutes, the ambulance arrives, loaded with paramedics ready to help. They speedily do a couple of checks and connect Christina to oxygen, which has an immediate effect. A man then lifts her from the couch onto the flatbed. Once she is strapped, they hastily wheel her into the ambulance. Sweet Mother jumps into the back of the ambulance and sits right beside Christina, panicking like a spring chicken. The driver takes off and shoots straight to Mercy Seed Hospital, which is located approximately twenty minutes away without traffic (if you were a regular motorist, so to speak).

As you may already know, emergency vehicles tend to go a whole lot faster because they have the right to speed, everyone yields to them, and they are allowed to run red lights. During the ride, Christina can't help herself. She is in so much pain and crying so hard, but at the same time, the paramedics have important questions to ask her. They need answers in order to help her accordingly. They notice her stomach extending and getting harder by the minute as it takes on a very weird shape during the ride to the hospital. Basically, her stomach is distended.

"Who is your doctor? When was the last time you felt your baby move? How far along are you?" Those and a host of other questions are being thrown at her one after the other. She tries her best to provide responses, and Sweet Mother is also helping with some answers as much as she can.

Approximately fifteen painful minutes later, they are at the premises of Mercy Seed Hospital. Christina is wheeled straight into the theater room. It is filled with so many doctors all dressed in green scrubs and disposable white net hats. Her doctor is in a delivery, so the other doctors have to step in and take care of her. The first thing they notice as they look at her is her distended stomach. They scan her stomach and discover her placenta has ruptured and completely detached from the uterus. The baby doesn't have a heartbeat. Another lady doctor opens Christina's mouth, examines it, and screams, "She is getting pale. We have to hurry up!"

In actuality, the doctors are all working at the speed of light, but considering Christina's condition and how pale she appears, this doctor feels like they could do better, as every single second is so critical in this moment. She fears they might lose Christina if they don't hurry up.

One of the male doctors turns to Christina and informs her that the baby has been compromised and they need to perform an emergency C-section. In all the pain and tears, Christina smiles and nods her head in approval, thinking she will have her baby soon. For some reason, she only hears that her placenta has ruptured and misses the part about her baby having been compromised.

As a matter of fact, she doesn't understand what a ruptured placenta implies and has no clue that all the speed with which the doctors are operating right now is to save her life. In hindsight, it is a good thing that she didn't quite comprehend what had been communicated to her. With her blood pressure already measuring so high in that moment, a full comprehension of the circumstances may have worsened the situation. Her blood pressure is too high for anesthesia to be administered. The doctors monitor it closely to act as soon as they can catch the right level. During this period, Christina throws up.

As a quick reminder, this is the first time she has thrown up since finding out she was pregnant. Fortunately, right after this vomit episode, an opportunity with an acceptable blood pressure level presents itself, and the medical team jumps right on it. They administer the anesthesia, perform the surgery, successfully deliver a stillborn baby boy, and save Christina's life.

A few hours later, Christina wakes up in the recovery room. She opens her eyes, and the first thing she spots is her dear Sweet Mother sitting on a small brown chair next to her bed with a wretched look on her face. The room looks peculiar to her. She notices a lot of tubes connected to her. She looks up to see where all the tubes are coming from and notices bags filled with blood and other liquids hanging on an IV stand by her headboard. She is a little confused. Recollecting her thoughts, Christina remembers she is at the hospital. She looks down and realizes that her big belly, though still big, has reduced significantly. This entire discovery happens in a split second.

"They delivered the baby!" she exclaims with a big grin on her face. Turning around, she locks eyes with Sweet Mother, who is now standing close to the bed, holding her hand. "How is the baby doing? Is it a boy or a girl?" Christina inquires.

Sweet Mother looks rather gloomy as tears drip from her eyes.

"What's the matter, Sweet Mother? Why are you crying?" Christina asks.

"You didn't hear?"

"Hear what?" Christina asks.

Sweet Mother moves even closer to Christina's bed, holding her hand tighter. Before she even utters a word, Christina starts having the feeling there is bad news. The look on her mom's face alone drives her to tears.

"I'm so sorry, babe. I thought you heard what the doctors said after they did the scan. I'm so sorry. It was a boy—a beautiful boy—but he didn't make it. I'm sorry."

Christina is horrified and speechless. All she can do is cry and cry and cry some more. She is crying so loud that people can hear her in the hallway. The nurses come rushing in to console her. They tell her all kinds of elevating tales, but nothing helps. Christina cries uncontrollably. She hurts deeply and feels inexplicable pain.

One after the other, the nurses exit the room—all except for one. Her name is Amanda. She is kind, gentle, soft-spoken, and filled with a lot of love, care, and compassion. She is Christina's nurse for the night. She grabs a chair and sits close to Christina's bed.

Wiping Christina's tears with one hand and holding her hand with the other, she says, "Would you like to see your baby now? He is so beautiful. He has a lot of hair on his head. He is beautiful."

"Is he alive?" Christina asks as she sobs underneath her oxygen mask.

"Unfortunately, he is not. I'm so sorry. But trust me; he is so beautiful. Let me bring him to you," replies Nurse Amanda.

Christina sternly rejects the offer. She is seriously infuriated. "I've told you I want to see my baby alive, not dead. What part of that do you not understand?" she snaps at Nurse Amanda.

"I'm sorry, Christina."

There is a long silence. Christina turns her head away from Nurse Amanda's direction.

"Get some rest. I will come back later to check on you," says Nurse Amanda in a very polite tone as she exits the room.

Shortly after Nurse Amanda leaves, another nurse comes in with news that Christina's room is ready. They will be moving her from the recovery room to the intensive care unit (ICU) where she will continue to receive medical care. It's a much bigger room with a much-needed bed for Sweet Mother. Poor thing—she has been on a hard and uncomfortable chair all along.

While in the ICU, Nurse Amanda once again brings up the idea of bringing the baby to Christina but is met with a lot of resistance—this time even more cruel than before. Sweet Mother, on the other hand, is doing a lot of thinking. She wants to find a good way to talk Christina into seeing the baby. Not only is she a mom, but she is a medical doctor. From the mom side of the spectrum, she understands the importance and closure that comes with seeing the baby, and from the medical side of it, she understands that a corpse does change with time. She knows it is important for Christina to see the baby before he starts changing. She would prefer Christina to remember this baby as fresh as he still is.

She tries to talk Christina into seeing the baby a couple of times with no success, but that doesn't stop her. She is determined to try again, each time using different strategies to talk to Christina. Finally, Christina gets to the point where she agrees to see the baby.

Sweet Mother presses the button, and almost instantly, Nurse Amanda walks in. It so happened that she was right around the corner doing her night duty runs.

As soon as she enters the room, Sweet Mother turns to her and says, "The baby please … You can bring him now."

Nurse Amanda takes a peep at Christina, who smiles and nods her head in approval. She smiles back at Christina, gives her two thumbs-up, and races out to fetch the baby. While she is gone, Sweet Mother assists in raising Christina's bed to an upright position, comfortable enough for her to sit and receive the baby once the nurse returns. A few moments later, the door opens, and they notice a stroller making its way into the room being pushed by Nurse Amanda. Christina and Sweet Mother are both teary. It's hard not to cry. Nurse Amanda gets teary too. She gives Christina a big hug, wipes her tears away, takes the baby out of the stroller, and hands him over to her.

The baby is nicely wrapped in a comfy white cloth with a blue and white hat on his head. Nurse Amanda helps unwrap the cloth from the baby's body, and Christina goes skin to skin with him, hugging him as tightly as she can and shedding buckets of tears. He is so beautiful and feels nice and warm. For a second, she believes he is alive. She opens his eyes and puts her head on his tiny chest, hoping for a heartbeat. If she could breathe life into her baby, she would.

Nurse Amanda leaves the room so Christina and Sweet Mother can have some private time with the baby. Simply put, they cry more tears before Nurse Amanda comes back to take him away. She tells Christina that whenever she feels like seeing him, she should let her know, and she will bring him up immediately.

CHAPTER 4

Delivering the News

While Christina is undergoing surgery, her mom is left with the task of informing Tim and the rest of the family about the tragedy. She is completely discombobulated. She can't understand how a perfect pregnancy has suddenly become a crisis. How will she break such tragic news to Tim? How will she break it to the rest of the family? Her heart is heavy, but she has to be strong. She must deliver the news somehow. She feels this big weight on her shoulders that translates into a feeling of helplessness.

After a long struggle, she picks up her phone, stares at it, and throws it back into her pocketbook before standing up and pacing around. She hears her phone ringing as she paces up and down the hallway. The sound of it makes her heart sink. Her first impression is that it may be Tim. She is shaking enormously as she scours her pocketbook for her phone. She finally reaches the phone, pulls it out, and looks at the caller ID, and realizes it is Christina's Dad calling. She breathes a sigh of relief as she clicks the answer button, dashing to a quiet corner for some privacy.

"Hello."

"Hi, honey. How is Christina doing?"

"I haven't seen her yet, honey, but the doctors say she is in a stable condition."

"OK. I'm on my way. I will be there in about fifteen minutes."

"Great! See you shortly."

She feels better just by learning that her husband is on the way. "As soon as he gets here, I will have him make the calls," she says to herself.

As she waits, she peeks at the clock from time to time, hoping for the fifteen minutes to elapse. Because she is so nervous, confused, and impatient at the moment, the clock appears to be moving slower than usual. She checks her wristwatch and mobile device just to make sure the wall clock is accurate, and to her greatest dismay, the time is consistent on all three devices. She decides to take a trip to the restroom in order to kill some time, but that's not helping either. Fifteen minutes feels like a lifetime. After what felt like an awfully long wait, fifteen minutes finally elapses. She changes seats and positions herself so she has a better view of the door in order to spot her husband the moment he walks through.

A few minutes later, her phone rings. She looks at the caller ID and picks it up saying, "Hi, honey. Are you here?"

"Hello, ma'am … emmm … This is Veronica from the clinic. I heard about what—"

Before she even states the purpose of the call, Sweet Mother interrupts in a disappointing voice. "Veronica, I'm going to cut you short because I can't talk right now. OK? Talk to you later."

She actually thought it was her husband calling when she picked up the phone. Although she had taken a look at the caller ID, somehow *Veronica* seemed like *Hubby* to her. Her stress level is transparent through her actions and reactions. She looks at the clock and realizes her husband is five minutes late. As she is about to dial his number, one of the doctors interrupt her to give a brief update on Christina and her situation.

"Ma'am, I'm Dr. Grover, one of the doctors who operated on Christina. I'm here to inform you that her surgery went well, and she is now in the recovery room."

"Oh! What great news! Can I see her now?" asks Christina's mom, quickly standing.

"Sure! But let me brief you on the surgery before you see her," replies Dr. Grover.

"Do you mind if I just lay eyes on her before you brief me please?" asks Christina's mom.

"You could, but I'd rather brief you first," replies Dr. Grover.

"Let me see her please … Please, Dr. Grover."

"OK. Come with me then," says Dr. Grover as he leads the way.

Christina's mom follows right behind him, walking as fast as she can in her high heels. (The fun fact here is that she loves her high heels. The only time you maybe can catch her in anything other than five-inch heels is when she is crawling out of bed, so as you can clearly see, the chances are very slim or even nonexistent. I mean, who travels on long-haul flights in heels? Anyway, that's a story for another day. Let's focus on Christina's recovery before we go off at a tangent.)

As they walk into the room, Sweet Mother is unable to come to terms with what she is seeing. Christina is lying in bed motionless with all sorts of monitoring devices connected to her. There is an oxygen mask over her face, a blood pressure cuff attached to her arm, an oximeter on her finger, plastic intravenous (IV) bags, and all sorts of tubes hanging from the five-leg stainless steel IV pole, all connected to Christina. Some of the IV bags are filled with blood, and some are filled with clear fluid; all of them dripping slowly through the tubes into Christina. There is a heart monitor with lines or tracings moving across the screen with wires running from it to Christina's chest. There is also a urinary catheter connected to Christina's lower body parts.

Being a medical doctor herself, she has a good understanding of what a patient in the recovery room following major surgery might look like. She also understands what all the equipment, wires, tubes, IVs, screens, and so on are used for. But, because the patient in recovery is her baby girl, her brain is processing things a little different at the moment. There has been a swift shift from doctor mood to parent mood without her realizing it. Everything in the room appears foreign and scary to her.

"Is she OK?" questions Sweet Mother.

"Yes, ma'am ... Yes, she is very stable and recovering nicely from the anesthesia. We are also making sure that she gets the best care possible. She is fine, ma'am," replies the nurse.

Sweet Mother doesn't seem convinced. Staring at the sack of blood hanging on the IV pole, she asks in a very low voice, "And the blood ... What's that for?"

"Let me take it from here while you stay back and keep watch over Christina," interrupts Dr. Grover.

The nurse nods her head in approval. Dr. Grover opens the door and turns to Sweet Mother. "After you, ma'am."

As they walk toward Dr. Grover's office, Sweet Mother's phone rings.

This time, it is actually her husband. *Finally!* she thinks. He is already in the building trying to find her.

"Hold on, honey. Let me talk to the doctor quickly," she says to her husband. She then lifts her head toward Dr. Grover. "Dr. Grover, my husband is in the building trying to find his way here. Can you please help with directions on how to get here if you don't mind?"

"Absolutely!" replies Dr. Grover.

"Here … He is on the line," says Sweet Mother as she hands over her phone to Dr. Grover. In less than five minutes, her husband joins them. He was just around the corner the entire time, but with many identical hallways in the labor and delivery unit, it was a little challenging for him for find his way. Dr. Grover briefs them on the surgery. He begins by highlighting the fact that Christina is lucky to be alive.

"Very few patients make it alive in such situations. She is a fighter, and you should be very proud of her and grateful for her life," says Dr. Grover.

By this time, all kinds of emotions are taking control of Christina's parents. They are absolutely stunned by Dr. Grover's words. They look lost and frozen as tears roll down their cheeks. Dr. Grover hands them tissues, gives them a moment to feel their emotions, and then continues by saying, "You know, Christina lost a lot of blood—almost all of her blood if I'm being completely transparent with you. When the abruption occurred, all the bleeding was internal, so no one could have seen signs of a bleed. All the blood remained inside of her, and that explains why her stomach was distended, out of shape, and rock-hard by the time she arrived here.

"When we performed her surgery, we took out a massive blood clot measuring three times larger than the size of a placenta, and she is still alive. She is a strong girl, you know. She is such a fighter. She is currently receiving a blood transfusion, including blood platelets and fresh frozen plasma (FFP), to replace her blood and liquid loss and help with her platelet count as well as her regulatory proteins and clotting factors. So far, she is responding nicely, I guarantee you.

"We are not yet sure of the cause of the abruption, but we will let you know once we find out, and we will include every detail in her medical report as well. Her room is also ready in the ICU, and as soon as she wakes up, she will be transported upstairs. There, we've got an excellent team who will provide her with outstanding care." He throws some more medical jargon around as he tries to shed more light on the situation. and reassures them that their daughter will be fine and then walks them back to Christina's room so they can be by her side.

The advantage here in being medical doctors is that they can get a good grasp of the report presented by Dr. Grover, which gives them a clear understanding of the severity of their daughter's situation. Although they believe she will pull through, they are still on pins and needles because they know exactly what it means to be unable to make your own blood. There is silence in the room as they all quietly process the circumstances they are now faced with.

Christina's dad breaks the silence first by clearing his throat. He turns to his dear wife and asks, "Hey, darling, have you spoken to Tim since the incident occurred?"

Lips tight and folded inward, she shakes her head from left to right, meaning she hasn't.

"I think now that we know what the situation is, we can give him a ring and keep him in the know," says Christina's dad.

Let me step outside and try to get in touch with them." As he walks out the door, he is thinking about how much he hates to be the bearer of bad news, but he has to man up and get it done.

In his many years in medicine, he has had to tell countless people that their loved ones have passed away, but it doesn't make this situation any easier on him. He paces around, trying to rehearse a line to say once he gets Tim on the phone, but nothing seems to sound right. After a few paces up and down the hallway, he finally bites the bullet and rings Tim. On the third ring, he picks up the phone excitedly. He has no idea that a bombshell is about to be thrown at him. Christina's dad goes straight to the point and delivers the news. As anticipated, Tim takes it hard. Christina's dad stays on the phone with him and calms him down, assuring him that Christina is recovering just fine and as soon as she wakes up, he will call back so he can speak to her.

"Did you get him?" asks Sweet Mother.

"Yeah, he is completely devastated! He is trying to see if he can catch the next flight to Baltimore, but looking at the time, he might only be able to leave tomorrow if he's lucky. Poor thing! He wants to speak to his wife so badly."

CHAPTER 5

Hospital Stay Highlights

Almost every nurse and doctor coming in and out of Christina's room mentions at least one of these words: red blood cells, white blood cells, platelets, or plasma. They seem concerned about the low numbers and appear to be in desperate desire to see these numbers on the rise. They are constantly testing, monitoring, measuring, and comparing results to see if there is any progress.

What are these things anyway? What role do they play in the human anatomy, and how important are they? Christina wonders.

All she understands at this point is that she has lost some blood and is getting a blood transfusion. She doesn't know how severe the situation is and isn't skilled enough to understand most of the terminology she hears the doctors and nurses throwing around in her room.

Blood carries oxygen and nutrients to the tissues and organs in our bodies and also removes waste products from it. Blood, as simple as it sounds, is actually made up of several components, including red blood cells, white blood cells, platelets, and plasma, each having its own very important role to play. Red blood cells carry and release oxygen throughout the body, while white blood cells form part of the immune system and help fight infections. Platelets help forming blood clots to stop bleeding, and plasma is a liquid in which the blood cells are suspended. Plasma also contains proteins partly responsible for blood clotting and globulins that help fight infections and diseases.

Evidently, without oxygen and nutrients, our body tissues and organs will shut down, and we will die. Losing large amounts of blood quickly can lead to serious complications, including death. The doctors and nurses involved in Christina's care are so concerned about her numbers because she has suffered severe blood loss, and they understand the consequences. Her bleeding is internal and severe. All the blood she lost remained inside her body, leading to swelling and pain. Remember the distended stomach and all the pain she experienced? It was due to all the blood that had accumulated inside of her.

To give us an idea of the severity of her situation in everyday language, Dr. Grover had mentioned that the blood clot inside of Christina was three times larger than the size of a placenta. A quick Google search tells us that in humans, the placenta averages 22 centimeters (9 inches) in length and 2.5 centimeters in thickness and weighs approximately 500 grams, which is slightly over 1 pound. Do you get the picture? We are talking about a blood clot that was 27 inches long and 3 inches thick and that weighed in at approximately 3 pounds. By simply trying to visualize this, my vision gets blurry. To think this actually happened to Christina is unbelievable.

The doctors and nurses continue to work assiduously, and Christina continues to receive medications to help stimulate her body to produce more blood cells. A few days later, the treatment starts to kick in, and her body slowly begins making its own blood cells. This is terrific news for her health care team. They are thrilled to see this progress. It's been a very bumpy couple of days filled with more lows than highs. They've worked tirelessly day and night in order to achieve these results and have every reason to be ecstatic. They continue to monitor her progress for one more day and are very happy with what they are seeing. Christina is responding to treatment nicely. They can now comfortably move her from the ICU into the labor and delivery unit where she will continue to receive medical care.

Christina's momr is beginning to lighten up. Being a medical doctor, she had a good understanding of what was going on the entire time but didn't say a word. Hearing those numbers and having a full comprehension of the ramifications were cutting her deeply. The health care team only knows her as Christina's mom. They have no idea that she is a medical doctor. They get in the room and throw medical parlance around thinking it's all coded and completely shielded from Christina and her mother. Turns out it was only shielded from Christina. Even when Christina's dad called or visited, Sweet Mother would give him updates in medical parlance. Christina had no chance of tapping into the severity of her situation, which was a good thing for her. Like the saying goes, what you don't know can't hurt you.

As they move into their new room in the labor and delivery unit, they notice that there is a sign on the door: an open palm with roots inscribed on it. They inquire and are told it's a sign to notify all caregivers and other hospital staff that the patient in the room has suffered infant loss so that they can be mindful of how they approach the patient. Brilliant idea! While Christina is getting used to her new health care team, she misses the ICU team. They were so kind and worked with every fiber of their being to make sure she was well taken care of.

The team in labor and delivery is equally as good—everyone is showing so much love, care, and compassion to her and her mother. Christina bonds with one particular caregiver by the name of Spikey. She is a Certified Nursing Assistant (CNA) and a little bit on the older side with a thick Southern accent. She's been with the hospital for thirty years. This woman loves her job—or at least she acts like she does.

Christina and her mom cannot understand why one would choose to be a CNA for that long and be so proud of it. A lot can be achieved in thirty years if you work at it. This woman could have gone to school to be a nurse or even a doctor in all these years. Christina and her mom are not in a place to judge, as she has no idea why this lady has stayed a CNA for thirty years. She can only appreciate her dedication to her patients and her love for what she does.

All along, Christina's mom hasn't been able to let any caregiver give Christina a bath. She is very particular and has been bathing her by herself since the incident. Spikey comes with a different touch. She wins them over almost instantly. She even succeeds in talking Sweet Mother into letting her give Christina a bath. Everything about Spikey seems authentic. She takes care of Christina as if she were her own daughter. She has a heart of gold. This family loves Spikey, and what's even more enchanting about her is that she stays consistent throughout Christina's stay at Mercy Seed Hospital.

The Rotten Apple

From the onset of the unfortunate event, Christina's mom has not left her room. She has dropped everything in her life to be with her baby. Christina feels so sorry for her mom and really wants her to take a break, even for one day. She sweet-talks her mom into going home for a couple of hours, and Sweet Mother reluctantly accepts. However, this turns out to be the worst mistake ever. The one day that she leaves Christina by herself, there is a disaster. Christina's nurse for the day is the absolute worst.

With Christina being in a delicate situation, you'd think every caregiver would show her some compassion or at least try to pretend to do so. But that is not the case here. This nurse is a total disaster. She is very well informed about Christina's situation but chooses to be inconsiderate, nasty, and rude. She refuses to give Christina her pain medication, bring her food, or readjust her on the bed and even yells at Christina when she asks for her pain medication.

The Head Nurse (also called a Charge Nurse) happens to be passing by and overhears a conversation between Christina and the rotten apple (nurse). She hears Christina crying and pleading with this nurse to give her medications, and not only is this rotten apple denying doing so, but she is equally becoming verbally abusive to Christina. That's crossing the line. The Head Nurse is not happy with what she is hearing. She rushes into the room right after the rotten apple leaves and finds Christina on her bed lying helplessly and crying for her Sweet Mother. She consoles Christina, nicely props her up in bed, calls the kitchen to bring her something to nibble on, and hands her medications. She proceeds to replace the rotten apple with immediate effect, and the lovely and caring new nurse continues to provide exceptional care to Christina for the rest of the day. Christina receives her food, medications, and other on-demand care in a timely manner, just the way it should be.

This encounter leaves Christina wondering if all the good care she got before was because the nurses were afraid of her mom or because they truly cared about her and her circumstances. She is gobsmacked. It's something worth thinking about.

Two days later, Christina is sitting in an upright position in her bed, and her Sweet Mother is sitting by her bed and telling her uplifting stories as usual. Soon, they hear a knock on the door, and a gentleman walks in with four others behind him. They all look like there is an emergency.

"Good morning, Ms. Christina."

"Good morning, sir. How may I help you?"

"I am the housekeeping supervisor, and my name is Wayne. Has your room been cleaned today by any chance?"

"No, it hasn't been cleaned yet."

"What about your bed?" he asks. "Have the beddings been changed?"

"No, but don't worry about it. My bed is not soiled. They change it if it gets soiled, and my mom and I have been doing a great job managing it."

"Ms. Christina, henceforth, your room and your bathroom will be cleaned every day, and your beddings will be changed every day as well. If no staff shows up to do the job, please let us know. As a matter of fact, I don't know why this hasn't been done from the get-go. I really apologize for that, ma'am." Pointing to the crew behind him, he says, "This is part of the housekeeping team who will be making sure your room is cleaned every day."

"Thank you, Wayne," Christina says.

"No, ma'am, thank you! We are here for you," he tells her. "Do you mind if they clean it right away?"

"Absolutely not," she says. "Go ahead."

Wayne places a paper behind the door, issuing a stern warning to his team. "I need you all to sign your names on here whenever you clean this room. Am I clear?"

"Yes, sir," they all reply.

This is a little weird. They've been in the hospital for days, and no special attention has been given to cleaning the room or changing beddings. The room isn't dirty either. Sweet Mother makes sure it always stays clean and sanitary. Not long after that, the nurses start coming in one after the other asking similar questions, including but not limited to: Are you OK? Did they bring your food yet? Have they given you your pain pills? When was the last time you had one? How is your pain? Are you comfortable?

Granted, they did regular checks, but for the length of time they've been at the hospital, the nurse assigned to her for the day was the only one who came in to check on her (with the exception of the Head Nurse who stood up for Christina when the rotten apple was being abusive). Every day, the assigned nurse will come in whenever her pager goes off or whenever she has to pass out medications. All these random checks by multiple nurses within a short interval are completely new and absurd. To crown it all, three doctors come in back-to-back … again, to check on Christina. How weird is this?

As they walk in and out of the room, one thing that is unanimous with all of them is that before leaving the room, they all say, "Please let us know if you need anything. We are here for you."

It almost sounds rehearsed, and Sweet Mother and Christina are in bewilderment. Sweet Mother asks one of the doctors what is going on and why so many checks all of a sudden.

In response, he smiles and says, "Oh nothing, ma'am. It's our job to make sure you are very comfortable here."

In actuality, the word was out. They had come to the realization that Christina's parents are prominent doctors in Maryland and are affiliated with many hospitals in the area, including Mercy Seed Hospital. From this point onward, Christina begins and continues to receive first-class care until she is discharged.

As much as the care and detailed attention are appreciated, Christina is struggling inwardly. She can't seem to comprehend why she is receiving more and better care just because the health care team is now in the know of who her parents are and what they do for a living. She finds this despicable and has a lot of unanswered questions regarding this scenario to date.

CHAPTER 6

Facing Reality

There are certain things that cannot be avoided when faced with them. Whether we like it or not, we have to deal with them at some point. The bitter truth is that Christina and Tim's baby cannot be refrigerated forever. Someday, his mortal remains will have to be disposed of. However, the couple is not thinking about this just yet. Christina is still in her sick bed fighting to get better. She hasn't quite processed the demise of the baby.

One gloomy afternoon, she is quietly lying in bed, listening to some mindfulness music. Nurse Lauren comes knocking at the door. She has to have a serious, uncomfortable and very important conversation with Christina.

"Hi, Christina."

"Hi, Nurse."

"My name is Lauren, and I'm here to talk to you about some options you have regarding your baby's funeral," she explains.

"Funeral? What do you mean?" Christina asks.

"Well, the hospital can do the funeral for you, or you can choose to do it by yourself. If you choose to go with the hospital, it is free of charge. You can also choose to attend or not to attend … It's entirely up to you to choose what works for you and what you are comfortable with. There will be other families there, so it might be a good way to bond with people who are experiencing the same loss. On the other hand, if you choose to do it by yourself in a more private setting with just you and your family in attendance, it will cost you some money—say, about $3,000 or so. Which option is better for you?"

Christina starts breaking down. She can't believe she is going through all of this. Lauren tries to console her to no avail and ends up rescheduling the talk, which gives Christina a day to think about the options.

The next day Lauren comes back. Just seeing Lauren makes Christina cry. She knows exactly why Lauren is there. She's had some time to discuss the options with Tim, and they have agreed on giving the hospital the go-ahead to proceed with the funeral.

"So, have you guys thought about the options yet?" Lauren asks.

"Yeah, we did," Christina says. "We've actually decided on what we want to do. We think we will have the hospital do it for us."

"Wonderful! That's a great choice. Will you be attending the ceremony?"

"If I've been discharged by then, yes, we will."

"Oh yes, you will be discharged by then. Our next ceremony will be coming up in two months, and I'm pretty sure you will be out of here by then," Lauren explains.

"Great! We'll be there."

"Perfect. I will need to go over some paperwork with you, and I would like you to sign some documents in order for me to proceed."

"Sure, go ahead."

In the process of going through the paperwork, Christina is not comfortable with one element. All babies who have passed away within the past few months (three to four months I believe), will all be placed in one large casket and buried together. This does not sit well with Christina.

"How many babies are there in total?" Christina asks.

"About forty," replies Lauren.

"Forty babies?" Christina echoes.

Lauren nods her head. Christina is in total shock. She imagines her baby with thirty-nine other babies in one casket and bursts into tears.

"I can't do this, Lauren. I can't. That's cruel and horrifying," says Christina as she cries.

"I take it you will be doing it by yourself then?" inquires Lauren.

"I need some time alone please. Come back later. Will you? Please come back later," says Christina.

"Sure I will. See you later this afternoon," Lauren says and exits the room.

Christina calls and updates Tim on the new shocking and disturbing findings, and they decide it will be best for them to have a private funeral for their baby. The thought of having their baby with thirty-nine others was repugnant to them. They knew they couldn't live with it and believed their baby deserved better.

Lauren shows up later in the afternoon and goes over the procedure of doing a private funeral. Christina is okay with it and signs the papers, agreeing to go private. As Lauren leaves the room, Christina feels so relieved. A huge burden has been lifted off her shoulders, and she strongly believes they've made the perfect decision for their little one.

A couple of days down the road, Christina's numbers continue to improve but at a low rate. The doctors are not comfortable discharging her from the hospital. They continue to monitor her closely while encouraging her to take supervised short walks up and down the hallway multiple times a day to help with blood circulation. It takes another two days for her numbers to hit the long-awaited mark. The doctors and all the staff involved in her care are so happy. Finally, Christina can now be discharged. She and her family are happy as well. They have been looking forward to this day for quite a while.

The doctors complete and sign the discharge orders, educating Christina and her family on how to continue with in-home care while out of the hospital. Before discharging her, the doctors discuss their findings on what may have caused the placental abruption. Centered on the fact that Christina has never smoked, has never used drugs, doesn't have preeclampsia (hypertension), is well below the age of thirty-five, was pregnant with a singleton, hasn't had a placental abruption in the past, had no abnormalities in her uterus, and didn't experience trauma to the abdomen during the pregnancy, the incident was considered to be an unexplained placental abruption.

It's a mystery and it's frustrating, but no one knows why it occurred. It would have been helpful to have a full comprehension of the mishap in order to have some closure and to prevent it from happening in future pregnancies. But if the doctors can't find anything, they can't find anything.

With their discharge packet in hand, Christina and her family finish packing up their belongings, and as soon as they are ready to walk out of the door, Nurse Amanda shows up. Yes, Nurse Amanda from the ICU, the very pleasant, caring, and friendly Nurse Amanda. Remember her, right?

She comes carrying something like a box with both hands and a big broad bright smile on her face. "I hear you guys are leaving today," she says from about three meters away.

"Yes, we are. Isn't that exciting?" says Christina's mom.

"Sure is. I'm so happy for you guys," Nurse Amanda replies. "Hi, Christina."

"Hi, Nurse Amanda."

"I have something for you, and I hope you will like it," says Nurse Amanda.

"Oh really? That's very kind of you."

"I would like to show you in private if you don't mind."

"Not a problem."

They head back into the room and close the door behind them. Nurse Amanda opens the box, and Christina is blown away. She is in tears as she goes through the contents of the box—tears of joy, I mean. Nurse Amanda had secretly taken the initiative to do something absolutely amazing, heartwarming, and special for Christina. She had taken and printed out excellent photos of the baby in his best state right after he was delivered, she had cut a little bit of his hair and preserved in a small zip-top bag, and she had even taken foot- and handprints of the baby. She preserved the baby's wristband from the operating room with the exact time of delivery on it. She even wrote a poem and placed it inside the beautiful baby blue rectangular box. What a brilliant idea! Christina is in awe and cannot thank Nurse Amanda enough.

With tears rolling down her cheeks, she looks Nurse Amanda in the eye and says, "You are the best thing that has happened to me in this hospital, Nurse Amanda. You are a superstar! You are an absolute godsend! Thank you from the bottom of my heart. You have no idea how much this means to me. I will forever be grateful to you and for you for all you have done for me. Thank you so much."

Nurse Amanda smiles and gives her a big hug. As they continue to converse, Nurse Amanda drops another bombshell. August 4, 2014, had been her first day of work as a labor and delivery nurse, and Christina's delivery was her first. She had just completed nursing school. She further revealed that she was the one who had given the baby a bath and dressed him up. This is beyond Christina's comprehension. To think that Nurse

Amanda was that thoughtful and proactive on her first day of work as a nurse is incredible. Such a brilliant girl she is!

"Anyway, I just dashed down to hand the memory packet to you. I have to go back to work, but I will keep in touch," says Nurse Amanda.

"Thank you so much, Nurse Amanda," replies Christina.

As Nurse Amanda rushes back to work, Christina joins her family, and they head home with mixed feelings; they are sad to be returning without the baby, but they are happy that Christina has pulled through and has finally been discharged from the hospital. With heavy hearts, they find a way to rejoice because they understand that it could have been worse. At least they have Christina with them, and that's a big enough reason to be grateful and to give thanks to God.

CHAPTER 7

Back to Work

You'd agree with me that whenever death occurs in a family, grieving family members and friends are always there to support one another in one way or another. However, there comes a time when they all begin to return to their everyday routines. They can only take so much time off. It is no different in Christina's case. As much as her family loves being there for her, the time has come for them to resume their daily activities. Those who flew in from out of town have to fly back out, locals have to go back to work, children have to go back to school, and Tim, as well, has to go back to work.

Returning to work is not an easy task after experiencing a recent loss, especially an unexpected one. Tim has to return to the business world sooner than he would like to. That's part of life. He hasn't seen his coworkers in a while and has no idea how to comport himself once he sees them. Should he cry? Should he tell them the whole story? Should he be silent? He is not sure what to do and plans on going with the flow however it unfolds.

Seeing his coworkers exposes him to a lot of expressions of sympathy and, "Sorry for your loss, Tim," reminding him of his baby and bringing back all his memories of the unfortunate event. As difficult as it is to hear and deal with all these expressions, they are way better than no acknowledgments at all. He has a set of very supportive coworkers except for one or two insensitive or ignorant ones who do not understand the grieving process.

Slowly but surely, things are beginning to get back to normal at work for Tim. He still has a few bad days when he will break down and excuse himself from important meetings but not as much as before. Thankfully, almost everyone around him understands to an enormous extent what he is going through, and no one chastises him for his actions during this painful transitional period. They see how hard he is trying and how hard he is working even in his grief.

Given that he has a high-pressure job with many deadlines to meet and little or no room for mistakes, he has to be extra careful, and he does a pretty good job managing that. He has come to the realization that it is hard for him to concentrate and retain information in his grief. He is easily distracted these days, and it is very likely for errors to occur in such a state of mind. To mitigate this, he checks his work twice and asks a colleague to double-check to be sure it is error-free before he submits anything. It takes a while using this strategy to survive at work, but he eventually gets back to 100 percent.

CHAPTER 8

Funeral Plans

Planning a funeral for your baby is one of the most traumatic things any parent can go through. The thought of having to hold a funeral is something Christina and Tim are struggling with, but they have no choice. If you lose your baby after twenty-four weeks of a pregnancy, the remains must be buried or cremated. It is the law, and there is no way around it. Whether you hold a funeral service before the burial or cremation is entirely up to you. Given the fact that all this is new to Christina and Tim, they decide to take some time to think things through before making any decisions regarding the funeral.

Weeks upon weeks go by without any formal discussion on the topic. They find it difficult to talk about it. They never thought they would be burying their own child, especially one they never had the chance to spend time with, love on, and bond with outside of the womb. They are so heartbroken and emotionally drained.

Three weeks after Christina returns home from the hospital, she gets a phone call from Nurse Lauren. "Hi, Christina. This is Nurse Lauren from the hospital. Did I catch you at a good time?"

"Sure."

"I was calling to find out if you've decided on when you will be having the funeral for your baby."

"Oh! We haven't decided yet, but we will do so and let you know."

"Okay. Try to do it quickly because our shared funeral program has been scheduled for October 3, 2014, and you must make arrangements with the funeral home to pick up your baby before then. If not, he will be included in the mass funeral on October 3."

There is silence on the line as Christina tries to process the information Nurse Lauren has just given her.

"Hello … Christina, are you there?"

"Yeah, yeah, yeah! I'm here. Is it okay if I talk things out with my family and give you a call back?"

"No problem! Go for it. I will talk to you later."

Christina drops to the floor on her knees, head buried in her lap as she blubbers uncontrollably. Sweet Mother runs toward her almost instantaneously.

"What's the matter, Christina?" asks Sweet Mother.

"Lau … ren …" She tries to mumble a few words, but one can hardly understand what she is saying.

Sweet Mother is very patient with her and tries her best to calm her down before getting into the details of the phone call. She reassures Christina that everything will be okay and that they will be there for her no matter what.

Christina and Tim must face the monster. They have no choice at this point. If they want things done their way, this is the time to act. As they try to figure out a good date for the funeral, they have to consider family and friends who live out of state and have expressed that they would like to be present at the funeral. This means they need to give them advance notice so that they can plan.

The very next day Nurse Lauren calls again. "Hi, Christina. It's Lauren from the hospital. I have some updates for you."

"Updates?"

"Yes, I'm so sorry I gave you the wrong information yesterday. All babies for the mass funeral will be picked up this weekend in order to prepare their bodies for the funeral. If you haven't picked up your baby's body by then, I'm afraid he will be included in the mass funeral."

"Wait a minute! You lost me. Can you repeat what you just said?" Christina asks.

"Sure I can. What I'm saying is that I made a mistake when I called you yesterday. I didn't realize that the bodies of the babies for the mass funeral will be picked up this weekend. You have to make arrangements with a funeral home to come and pick up your baby's body before this weekend. If you go through the paperwork I gave you, you will find a lot of information about different funeral homes in the area and their contact information. You can get in touch with them, and I'm sure they will be more than happy to help you. We work with them, and they are very professional."

"OK … thank you."

"Please call me back and let me know which funeral home you've selected and when they will be here," Lauren says.

"Will do."

"Have a great day, Christina."

"Thank you."

Christina gets off the phone and calls Tim immediately, but unfortunately, Tim doesn't pick up his phone. "Pick up!" Christina screams in frustration, stamping her feet on the ground. She tries a couple more times in total desperation to no avail. She is so confused and infuriated. She runs upstairs, heading straight for the stack of papers they had brought home from the hospital. She has never gone through any of these documents since they'd come back home.

"I can't do this!" she exclaims in tears. "Why me? Why? Why me?! Help me, Lord!" Christina laments as she goes through the documents.

Just then, the doorbell rings. It's Sweet Mother. Christina reluctantly heads for the door, wiping her tears away in an effort to conceal her current situation, but it's still obvious she's been crying. Her eyes are red, and her face is dull and a little on the pink side.

"Hey, babe, you've been crying again. What's going on?" inquires Sweet Mother.

"Nurse Lauren called," replies Christina.

"Oh no … not Lauren again. Why does she keep calling? What does she want? Didn't she call you yesterday?" Sweet Mother asks, standing by the door with both hands resting on her hips, her head slightly raised and eyes wide open. As she listens to Christina explaining the purpose of the call, her anger grows even larger. She's never been a fan of Nurse Lauren based on how she carries out her duties.

She fully understands that Nurse Lauren is doing her job, which, unfortunately, includes having uncomfortable and painful conversations with grieving patients, but at the same time, she believes that it could be done in a more careful, companionate, and condoning manner. But no—not with Nurse Lauren. She delivers her information in the rawest and strictest forms possible—no dilutions, no sugarcoating. She shoots straight to the point. Sweet Mother absolutely abhors this and qualifies it as total unprofessionalism.

Regardless of how emotional they may be or how distraught they may be with Nurse Lauren at this point, one thing is eminent—they have a situation that needs to be handled with immediate effect. They either put all emotions and frustrations aside and face the monster or let the hospital take control. There is a decision to be made here. Coming to this realization, they decide it is best to calm down, go through the documents, and get the information they need to proceed with the process of planning the funeral themselves.

As they go through the documents, Sweet Mother notices that Christina is really struggling. A lot of tears are rolling down her cheeks, and she is trying so hard to hold them back.

"Hey, babe, look at me," says Sweet Mother in a very soft voice, extending both hands toward Christina.

Christina slowly lifts her head and locks eyes with Sweet Mother. She looks so sad, pale, and miserable with tears prickling her eyes.

Holding Christina's hands and looking her straight in the eye, Sweet Mother utters, "Let me take care of this, OK? Get some rest, babe."

"Are you sure?" Christina asks.

"Anything for you, babe," replies Sweet Mother as she nods her head, smiling and patting Christina on the back. "Get some rest. If I need you, I will let you know," she adds.

"Thank you so much! Thank you, mom," Christina replies.

While Christina is getting some rest, Sweet Mother continues to go through the documents, gathering all the information she will need to help her make an informed decision. She also gets on the computer to research the recommended funeral homes in the area, eliminating those with not-so-good reviews. This helps narrow her search from a whole page of phone numbers to a select few that she feels are worth contacting. She calls them up one after the other before arriving at a final decision.

Out of the four funeral directors she speaks with, there is something about Mr. Sky. He is considerate and sensitive to her needs and requests and equally empathetic of her situation. Simply put, he handles the call with a lot of patience, compassion, and professionalism, which Sweet Mother greatly appreciates. Mr. Sky is the second person she calls, and as soon as she gets off the phone with him, she feels some peace and instantly knows that he is the right guy to work with during this tragic moment in their lives. She doesn't get this feeling with the other three funeral directors.

In the process of talking with these funeral homes, one thing is unanimous across the board: they will need to purchase a plot at the cemetery to use for the burial. This means she has to call the cemetery about purchasing a piece of land. Based on the rapport that she's built with Mr. Sky, she decides to give him a quick ring for more information on how to go about this. Mr. Sky recommends his top two cemeteries in the area, highlighting the one he would choose and why. The one he highly recommends happens to be close to home, which sounds like the perfect choice for this grieving family.

Sweet Mother discusses all her findings with Christina and Tim, and they decide to take a drive to both cemeteries in order to arrive at a final decision. After careful analysis and thoughtful considerations, they conclude that Angel Memorial Cemetery on Rosewood Road in Baltimore, Maryland, will be the best option. It is very close to home, the staff is amazing, and they find it very peaceful. They are confident and happy with their choice. They couldn't have chosen a better resting place for their little one. The next step is to purchase a plot in the cemetery where the baby will be buried.

As the family sits in the lobby brainstorming on other issues relating to the funeral, Ms. Yolanda approaches them to assist. She is the unit manager and family service counselor and will be the main point of contact during the entire process at Angel Memorial Cemetery. She is a pleasant and soft-spoken lady. She makes them so comfortable. It is evident that she has been doing this for a long time, loves her job, and is good at it. She explains the process to them in detail and sets out to take them on a drive to pick out a plot where the baby will be laid to rest.

Beneath the clear Baltimore skies, they drive behind Ms. Yolanda's car, which drives slowly through the nicely paved tracks with graves on both sides (something that really terrifies them). There is dead silence in the car, and the five-minute drive feels like a thirty-minute drive through the graveyard. Finally, they arrive at the section with available plots. As they shop around, Christina notices an indescribably long stretch of baby graves—way too long for one to see where it ends.

Some of the graves have gravestones and memorials on them, and some don't. As they walk along, Christina reads the memorials on the graves. Her focus is on the ages of these babies, and the oldest she notices lived for five months. She feels the pain of the parents of these babies and their families. It hurts her so much that she cries. On the bright side, she realizes that she is not alone. This walk is actually benefitting her psychologically.

"Look at all these baby graves," she says to herself as she looks around. "So many people have traveled down this path. I am not isolated in my tragedy. I am not alone. My baby will not be alone. He will be with all these little angels. They will be his friends." She smiles through her tears and continues the walk through the graves until they arrive at their destination in the cemetery.

As Ms. Yolanda is trying to show them the available plots while explaining the dimensions, Christina interrupts. "I will take the plot right after that new-looking grave if its available … please."

Everyone turns to Christina, and she has this big, broad smile on her face, which surprises them and leaves them wondering what caused the sudden change in her body language.

"Oh … This one, you mean?" Ms. Yolanda asks, pointing to the plot nearest to her.

"Yes," replies Christina with an even broader smile on her oval-shaped face.

"I think this might be taken, but give me a moment and let me double-check. I might be wrong," says Ms. Yolanda.

Hands trembling, she quickly reaches for her phone and pulls it out from the black oblong waist phone holder securely fastened to her belt and places a call (probably to the office). As soon as she gets off the phone, she turns straight to Christina with a disappointed but apologetic look on her face. "Sorry, Christina. I just confirmed that the plot you want is not available."

"Don't be sorry, Ms. Yolanda. It's totally fine. I will take the next one. Is it available?"

"Yes, it's available."

"Thank you! That's where our baby will be laid to rest then," says Christina.

"OK," replies Ms. Yolanda with two thumbs up at Christina.

They then drive back to the office, finish up the required paperwork, make the payment, and leave the premises, feeling so much better as one big item has now been scratched off their to-do list.

On their way home, they contact Mr. Sky (the soft-spoken funeral director) with an update on the plot purchase. Mr. Sky would like to set up a brief meeting with them to discuss the next steps in the process. Fortunately, his afternoon calendar is clear, and they both agree to a four o'clock meeting, which works perfectly. They drive straight to the funeral home for the meeting, arriving twenty minutes early, which leaves them with more than enough time to park the car, check in with reception, and get to Mr. Sky on time. Things work out perfectly, and a few minutes before four o'clock, Mr. Sky comes walking down the hallway leading to the reception.

"You must be Christina and Tim," he says.

"Yes," replies Tim. "And I reckon you are Mr. Sky?"

"You are correct. I am Mr. Sky! Very pleased to meet you all. Accept my condolences."

"It's OK. Meet my mother-in-law. She's helping us plan the funeral," Tim explains.

"Oh yeah, we've spoken a few times over the phone. Very nice to finally meet you, ma'am. My condolences," says Mr. Sky as he gives Sweet Mother a firm handshake.

"Nice to meet you too, sir, and thank you for your patience and for doing what you do. It takes a substantial amount of courage to constantly deal with people in grief. You are truly amazing," replies Sweet Mother.

"Thank you! And thank you for trusting us. Please come with me to my office and have a seat before we proceed," says Mr. Sky.

"The pleasure is ours," replies Sweet Mother.

Mr. Sky leads the way while Christina, Tim, and Sweet Mother follow right behind him. They walk past a few offices before arriving Mr. Sky's office. He makes them very comfortable before diving into the details of their services and what he can do for them to assist with the funeral process.

Deciding on everything surrounding a funeral arrangement is not an easy task to handle. Christina, Tim, and Sweet Mother are so grateful that Mr. Sky will be handling almost everything for them from this stage forward, including but not limited to the following:

o Taking care of all the necessary paperwork, including the certificate of stillbirth.
o Transferring their baby's body from the hospital to the funeral home.
o Taking care of the baby's body and preparing him for burial.
o Assisting in picking out a casket, headstone, and grave flowers if needed.
o Transporting the baby's body to the cemetery for the funeral.
o Directing the funeral.
o Providing a clergy if needed.
o Assisting with the funeral program if needed.

Evidently, having a good funeral director removes some of the legwork of having to handle some difficult and emotional tasks as listed above. This family feels so blessed to have such an incredible gentleman in Mr. Sky. He is willing to do more than his duties outline. He handles every single detail in the entire process with extraordinary professionalism and compassion. Sometimes, it's not about what you do but how you do it that matters. They leave Mr. Sky's office with a full understanding of how the entire process will be handled.

They all feel like a huge weight has been lifted off their shoulders. They can now relax, which is hard to do when you are in grief, knowing that their wishes will be respected and that their expectations will be met if not exceeded. As expected, Mr. Sky delivers on his promises, and the baby is finally laid to his final resting place on September 19, 2014, after an emotional but beautiful ceremony held in his honor.

CHAPTER 9

Agonizing Reminders

The days, weeks, and months following this loss are proving extremely difficult and painful for Christina, and that's understandable. On most days, she feels withdrawn and moody and can hardly concentrate or sleep during this troubled time. Feelings of anger, sadness, and confusion are present, and I think that's called grief, right? Sometimes the feelings seem to be more than she can handle. She is finding it hard to comprehend the fact that their baby is gone. The thought of it makes her want to scream, shout, kick, and cry out loud.

With painful reminders of the loss everywhere, it is hard for Christina to be OK. She is experiencing both emotional and physical trauma, and both are very insistent. While the emotional trauma is the worst kind of pain she has ever experienced, the physical is an equally ruthless and painful reminder.

There is this annoying enormous vertical cut on her still-protruding stomach with huge staples carefully placed over it. She sees this multiple times a day, and the cut is unbearably painful. If you have this massive painful incision on your belly and you turn around and see your bundle of joy lying in his or her basinet or crib right next to you, you embrace the pain and enjoy your baby. However, when there is no baby to cuddle and love on and you are dealing with all these physical changes and pain, how can you possibly keep it together?

The time Christina spent in the ICU is another agonizing reminder. She was in the ICU and on blood transfusion with depleted plasma and platelets. She had a catheter connected to her, she couldn't even bathe her own body, and she was unable to move herself from one position to the other or help herself out of bed. She had no strength to perform any physical activity, and her incision was still very fresh and distressing. Laughing and/or coughing were a nightmare due to the pain, and bending over was a huge challenge for her.

Lochia (vaginal bleeding) is also present. Although this is a normal process that occurs after a vaginal delivery or C-section as the woman's body is getting rid of the lining of the womb and blood from where the placenta was attached, this is all too emotionally painful for Christina. Sticking those enormous, highly absorbent pads into those hideous-looking disposable mesh granny undergarments would have been laughable in a good way if baby were here. Without baby, this activity shifts to a miserable, abhorred one.

A few days after the unfortunate event, Christina's breasts begin to feel large, tight, tender, and painful. It is breast engorgement, the process by which a woman's breasts fill with milk in the first few days after giving birth. She is mystified as to what is going on and absolutely livid at the realization that her breastmilk is coming in with no baby to breastfeed. She didn't envision this, so it's extremely emotionally distressing and feels unfair. Christina begins crying hysterically, wondering why baby isn't here to drink the milk.

Instead of feeding her baby, she is faced with learning how to suppress her breastmilk. Between applying ice packs and cabbage leaves to her breasts and taking pain killers, she is successful at finding some relief from the discomfort and diminishing the rate at which her breasts are filling up. But is this really a coveted activity after losing your baby? Wouldn't you rather be feeding your baby the breastmilk? Christina finds this brutal.

Her due date is another painful reminder—one that is inevitable and has the tendency to reignite grief over and over again. Approximately two weeks after the loss, Christina is confronted with a sad reminder as her actual due date arrives. She finds herself in a dark place, experiencing all sorts of intense emotions such as sadness, anger, pain, guilt, anxiety, frustration, loneliness, fatigue, depression, and a whole lot more that leave her reeling. She tries her best to control her emotions to no avail. There are all these vivid flashbacks of her entire pregnancy and the events of August 4, 2014. She remembers everything in great detail and is crying hysterically. It is really hard on her. The good news is that as the years go by, the yearly reminders begin to shift from a setback in her grieving process to reflections of how important her baby was to her.

Even when Christina begins to feel better physically and takes the chance to step out for some grooming activities, she encounters challenges.

She goes to the nail salon to get her nails done, and the ladies are so excited to see her. They have no idea she has lost the baby, so they proceed to ask her how the baby is doing. Another day she goes to the hair salon and encounters the same thing, and this time it's even worse, as her hair stylist comes hard at her with an insensitive question: "How could you not have known that your placenta was in danger? You should have gone to the ER immediately to save that baby's life." Wow! Did you just read that? Is this horrible or what? Christina can't take it and storms out of the salon with her hair half washed.

Approximately a week after the salon incident, she braves it again and walks into the bank to do make long overdue transactions. The teller is thrilled to see her with a diminished belly and with enthusiasm asks, "Oh wow! Congratulations, I see you've had the baby. How is he or she doing?"

Christina's face drops as she informs her that baby passed away. The teller sympathizes, apologizes for asking, and proceeds with the transaction. As she does, there is an awkward silence between them, and Christina can see the regret on her face for asking. But how would she have known about the loss Christina had suffered?

Even at church when people see her, they want to know how the baby is doing and whether she had a boy or girl. They look excited and happy for her without knowing that baby didn't survive. This continues to happen for a couple more worship sessions until the news gets around that she lost the baby.

One day Christina and her mom are at their local grocery store on Reisterstown Road in Owings Mills, Maryland, trying to stock up on some groceries while Christina benefits from a walk. It was a typical shoot-two-birds-with-one-stone situation, if you will. As they wheel their cart down the aisle, a sweet, soft-spoken lady walks up to them, hands them her babysitting services flyer, and begins to sell herself as a good babysitter, saying she will make an excellent choice for Christina's baby. At the time, Christina still has a protruding belly and appears pregnant.

A whole lot of these uncomfortable things continue to happen for a good while before tapering off. It's hard to get away from this stuff, you know. There are reminders everywhere. Even on the days she wakes up feeling really good, there is that one person who will say something that will remind her of their loss. For example, she is standing on the driveway catching some vitamin D when the mailman arrives all smiles in his mail truck and says, "It's been awhile, ma'am. How is baby doing?"

Then there are those people who won't stop questioning her. Christina wants to think they all mean well, but the constant probing frustrates her. She gets bombarded with questions: Where did this happen? How did it happen? Did you do an autopsy? What caused it? Were you checking your blood pressure? Did you do xyz test? What did your doctor say about it? It feels like a court session, and she is getting bored to death.

And then you have the sympathizers who cry at almost every phone call and talk about how they just can't believe the baby is gone. These people can't help themselves. They just can't bring themselves to talk about anything other than the baby's demise. Before long, Christina figures out how to deal with them. She just doesn't answer the phone when she sees their names flashing on her caller ID. She acknowledges their concern via text messaging, and it works better that way.

We almost forgot about those with constant pressure. They keep telling her to go ahead and get pregnant right away without trying to understand if it's even a possibility or something that Christina wants at this time. They say things such as, "It's been a month. What are you still waiting for?" Or, "I hope you've started trying to conceive already. Don't wait for too long."

And you've also got happy moments that are equally painful reminders, such as friends, family, and colleagues having healthy, beautiful babies. The baby shower invites keep coming in. In her pain, Christina has to shop for presents for babies and attend baby showers if she can and be happy for these other women.

She also keeps seeing cute babies wherever she goes. Left, right, and center—there always seems to be someone with a stroller pushing a little cutie pie around. Whenever she drives around, she can easily see those Baby on Board stickers proudly displayed on cars. These are all things she never really noticed before she suffered this loss. She also occasionally comes across babies with names she and Tim had considered for their baby.

She even meets this beautiful baby boy named Keith Richardson who was born on August 4, 2014. Baby Keith shares the same birthday as her stillborn angel. Christina sees her baby in this little boy. *So this is what my baby would have looked like by now if he stayed*, Christina thinks to herself. For some reason, baby Keith acts like he understands what Christina has been through. He places his cute little head gently on Christina's chest and stays in that position for a good while. Christina is comforted and establishes such a bond with this baby that she asks his mom if she could bring him a couple of times a week for a playdate. Keith is a painful reminder but one that ends up helping Christina heal. She loves this little boy.

With all of these things going on and with people expecting her to grieve in a prescribed manner, she constantly hides under her covers to cry whenever she can and does a lot of shower crying too. For the most part, her shower is her favorite crying spot because it offers the possibility to escape from people and just truly feel her emotions and express them through tears without feeling any guilt or pressure. The bathroom as a whole confers a measure of privacy, and the sound of falling water further masks the sound of her crying. This setting works well for Christina, as she is beginning to realize that it is advantageous not to flaunt her vulnerability anymore.

Moreover, whenever she emerges from a shower-cry session, she feels so much better, probably because showering and crying are both comforting activities in their own right. She finds that warm showers relax the muscles in her body and relieve tension, allowing her to feel an overall sense of comfort, calm, and peace.

CHAPTER 10

A New Page

Taking into consideration the events of August 4, 2014, and its aftermath and as advised by the doctors, Christina and Tim decide to give it a couple of years before trying again for another baby. The fear of an unexplained complete placental abruption is stuck in their minds. They fear it might happen again and do not want to go through the same kind of agony they've experienced. In that time, Tim secures a new job overseas. What a perfect distraction—something new and exciting to talk about!

In a couple of months, they will be relocating to Abu Dhabi, the capital city of the United Arab Emirates. They are so excited not only for the offer but also for the fact that they will have the opportunity to get away, leave all the pity parties and negative energy thousands of miles behind them, and focus on rebuilding themselves.

Fast-forward a few months, and the move finally happens. They now live in Abu Dhabi. Expat life in general is amazing. Abu Dhabi feels like a vacation, and they are making the most of it. A few months in, they are well settled and very conversant with their new environment. They decide to try for another baby. Six months down the road, Christina still hasn't fallen pregnant, and she is beginning to get troubled.

Initially, she believed they weren't trying at the right time in the first few months of the journey because Tim travels a lot for work. But things are beginning to take a different turn. Christina is beginning to wonder if something could be wrong with her system. *This is more than failing to try during the conception window of a woman's cycle*, Christina says to herself. She turns to the internet, hoping to find useful information as to why she is not getting pregnant. Unfortunately, she keeps stumbling on negative information from women who have been trying for years and years with no success.

This really scares Christina. She starts regretting her decision to turn to the internet for answers but still finds herself online in desperate need of that one positive piece of feedback to make her feel better. Eventually, she finds a few uplifting posts, but they are not exactly related to her situation.

More confused and terrified than she was when she first came to the realization that something might be wrong, Christina starts thinking of consulting a doctor to discuss her situation. She talks about it with her husband, and they agree that it is best to see a doctor. She would love to get a copy of her medical records to take to the doctors so they can best understand her history. Luckily, we live in a totally digital world, so Christina can have her records from her doctor's office back in the United States in no time.

With everything in hand, she begins researching a good ob-gyn in her area just like any reasonable person would do. After a few days and a whole lot of phone calls to hospitals and clinics, she compares notes and arrives at a decision as to which doctor to consult. She calls and takes the next available appointment for one o'clock the following afternoon.

For some reason, Christina wakes up the next day more energized than ever before, partly because she strongly believes today will mark the beginning of the end of the battle she's been fighting for the past six-plus months trying to get pregnant. She has also come to the realization that although it is OK to be optimistic, setting timelines on things you can't control can be very disappointing if desired outcomes are not met. With this analogy in mind, she promises herself to take things easy as she continues her journey trying to conceive.

She decides to go for a run, something she had enjoyed doing in the past. In a hurry, she slips into her sports gear and hits the pavement. According to Runstatic (a running app on her phone), she covered eleven miles in the space of an hour during that run. That's pretty impressive for a nonathlete. She returns home sweating profusely with her heart rate slightly raised. She feels super exhausted, but at the same time, she is proud of herself for the accomplishment. She jumps into the shower and takes a long, hot shower, singing periodically as she does so. She is in a very joyous mood.

At 11:30 a.m., her alarm clock goes off with a reminder to get ready for her appointment. She'd been advised to arrive a half hour early in order to fill out the new-patient paperwork. The hospital is only a seven-minute drive from home, and she has her clothes laid out, implying all she has to do is to get dressed and drive to the hospital, so she has plenty of time to play with. Some twenty minutes later, Christina is sitting in the car ready to go. She arrives at the hospital well ahead of time, finds a good parking spot, and heads to the main entrance where she is directed to the gynecology clinic located to the left of the facility.

After a two-minute walk, she spots a sign above a double-door entrance that reads: "Gynecology Clinic." She walks in and checks in with the receptionist who asks for ID and an insurance card before handing her the new-patient-information paperwork to fill out. It is so thick one would think she was about to sign her life away. She fills out the paperwork as accurately as she can and hands it back to the receptionist who then asks her to take a seat and wait to be called.

Finally, after a reasonable wait time, she is called to see the doctor. Christina walks in, and the doctor seems to either be in a rush or unsettled. *Maybe she is dealing with a messed-up schedule*, Christina thinks to herself. Trying not to be judgmental, Christina puts on a very positive attitude and smiles at the distressed-looking doctor, and they salute each other. The doctor offers her a seat and goes straight to the point.

"What brings you here today, my dear?" inquires the doctor.

"I am having issues getting pregnant, Doctor," replies Christina.

"How long have you been trying?"

"A little over six months now."

"Six months only? You haven't tried enough, darling. It's only been six months. Try again for another six months, and if you still do not get pregnant in that time, we will see what we can do. You are still very young. Go and keep trying. You will get pregnant," says the doctor.

"Doctor, can you at least run some tests today to make sure everything is OK?" Christina pleads.

"No, darling. I cannot. Go and try for six more months, and if no pregnancy occurs, come back and see us," replies the doctor.

Christina is appalled. She stares at the doctor with her eyes and mouth wide open and eyebrows slightly lifted as she tries to digest what the doctor has just told her.

The doctor breaks the silence by saying, "I know. Believe me, I do. It may feel like you've been trying forever, and maybe you have, but it's important to know that most couples do not conceive immediately." She continues by giving Christina some statistics. "About 80 percent of couples conceive after six months of trying. Approximately 90 percent become pregnant after twelve months of trying, assuming, of course, they have well-timed intercourse every month."

Christina finally finds her voice and responds by saying, "I thought people got pregnant by mistake. I was pregnant before, and we weren't even trying at the time. I found out after four weeks of marriage that I was pregnant. As you can see, I clearly do not fall in the 80 or 90 percent category." There is silence for some time. Christina is getting very emotional and teary.

"Don't worry. You will get pregnant. Just go home and keep trying. Give it some more time. I can't do anything right now," says the doctor.

Christina is trying to utter a few words, but the doctor cuts her off. "Look, darling, I really have to go. I just started working here last week, and I have so many meetings to attend. Have a nice day, darling." The doctor is packing up as she speaks.

Christina has never experienced anything like this before. She is in a befuddled state, but one thing she knows is that this is definitely not the doctor she would like to consult again. She thanks her and heads for the door, fully convinced this was her first and last time with this doctor. "What a waste of my precious time!" Christina mutters to herself. She hurries to her car and drives home aggravated.

The scenario at the doctor's office keeps playing in her mind and driving her imagination wild. Another six months of possibly waking up every twenty-three to twenty-four days (Christina's average cycle) to a period can be daunting for someone who is actively trying to get pregnant. Being new to the country makes it even more challenging, as she barely knows anyone to talk to. She hasn't made any friends yet. Her only source of information at this point is the internet.

The good thing is that regardless of the challenges, she doesn't falter.

She profoundly believes that if she intensifies her research, she will eventually find a good doctor. "I think I need to go out and catch the sunset while sipping on some hot tea," Christina says to herself. So far, she is in love with the Corniche, one of the best places for relaxation, fun, and entertainment in the city. It is the city's seafront promenade, which is packed with parks, fountains, cafes and restaurants, breathtaking gardens, and exotic distinctly shaped skyscrapers overlooking the sea with its clear-blue water and incredibly white sandy public and private beaches. Here, you'd find a community composed of a melting pot of nationalities, cultures, and identities.

She quickly changes into a beautiful floral maxi sundress, pairing it with white tongue sandals that complement the dress well. She lets her hair down, grabs a small cross-body bag that can only fit her wallet and mobile phone, takes one last look at herself in the mirror, and confirms her ensemble. (Generally speaking, she is a flamboyant dresser, and looking good is one of her outlets.)

As she grabs the car keys, something occurs to her. Parking at the Corniche is a severe pain in the neck. You spend so much time circling around trying to find a parking spot, and when you eventually do, it's usually so far off that you get discouraged by the distance you have to walk to arrive at your destination. Factoring all these annoyances in, Christina decides to catch a taxi. "It's only about 7AED ($1.90) anyway," she says to herself and walks to the closest taxi stand where she catches a cab.

Approximately ten minutes later, she is seated at a strategic corner on the terrace of her favorite café called Café Saba. From where she is sitting, she has a perfect view of the ocean and the city. The location is prime, the café is pristine, the weather is perfect, the skyline is changing, and the sun is about to set. She is surrounded by stunning, breathtaking views— exactly what the doctor ordered! Sitting under the lovely skies, she sips on some authentic lemon mint drink (a very popular and refreshing drink in the region) while listening to some Middle Eastern music as the waves gently lap the shore.

Life feels perfect again. She is gradually forgetting about the event at the doctor's office. She orders a seafood platter and some Moroccan mint tea—her favorite of all time. I'm sure you can tell she likes mint, right? She starts off with lemon mint, and now she is on mint tea. Sometimes when you travel, the flavors of certain foods and drinks of a country or city stay with you and play a big role in summing up your experience in a country. Authentic Moroccan mint tea is one of those flavors for Christina. She loves everything about this tea—from the way it is served to its flavor, its taste, and even its aftertaste. She loves it!

It is served in small glasses that may remind you of a juice glass or an overly generous shot glass, decorated in many different vibrant colors and patterns and placed on a coordinating tray. The tea comes in a bulbous-shaped silver teapot that is similar to the British Manchester with a long spout and a domed lid. It always feels like a Moroccan tea ceremony to Christina whenever she gets to drink this tea. Because Café Saba is the only spot where you will find this at the Corniche, this has become Christina's secret place whenever she needs to unwind while relishing what she calls authentic Middle Eastern hospitality.

The sun hasn't set yet; however, it is low on the horizon with a yellowish color. Her food has been served, and she is enjoying every bit of it. She notices one of the skyscrapers (whitish-silver in color) beginning to glow yellow and the sun bouncing off the other brown-colored building to the left, creating a bright reflection and reflecting the sun. Christina is in awe. She is enjoying the view and can't take her eyes off it. The streetlights are not on yet, and the sunlight is still bouncing off the clouds and sky.

A few moments later, Christina realizes that the sun has dropped farther below the horizon. Before she even blinks, the light is bouncing off the atmosphere above the skyscrapers, and the clouds are beginning to display an incredibly beautiful color. It gets brighter for about a quarter of an hour, and in that time, she watches the sunlight below the horizon bouncing off the clouds. It is beginning to appear darker. The pink in the clouds is slowly disappearing, and the sky is getting even darker, but this only lasts a few minutes as the lights from the skyscrapers begin to shine, overcoming the darkness. The sky gradually becomes beautiful with multiple colors. Coupled with the brightness of the streetlights, it forms a stunning reflection on the Corniche Bay. It's so dreamlike you would confuse it for a phantasmagoria.

In another few minutes, the sky becomes darker, and the whole Corniche begins to glow, creating a beautiful bright orange reflection in the bay. Within the twinkle of an eye, sunset is over. Christina is one happy lady; she enjoys catching the sunset whenever possible. That said, she asks for her bill, settles it, and catches a cab back home, feeling well invigorated. What an evening well spent!

The next day, she decides to continue her search for an ob-gyn, strongly believing there must be a good one out there. "One bad experience won't stop me. I won't give up," Christina murmurs to herself.

She makes several phone calls and finally secures a ten o'clock appointment with a doctor at Shamsa Hospital. While at her appointment, this doctor takes the time to learn about Christina, her medical history, and what brings her to the hospital. She portrays certain personal qualities, both emotional and physical, that resonate with Christina. There is this warm aura that surrounds this doctor. It is evident that she understands this is a vulnerable time in Christina's life.

Christina feels like this doctor personally understands what she is going through, and this makes her very comfortable. Not only has she found a gynecologist, but she's found one who also takes on the role of a counselor and a confidant, and that's exactly what she needs at this moment in time. Set up on Christina's medical history, the doctor wants to put in an order for some blood tests to be done in order to get a good understanding of what Christina's problem might be, if any. Unfortunately, there is a challenge.

These hormone panel tests can only be done during a certain window in a woman's cycle, and today is not a favorable day in Christina's cycle. She will have to come back on day two of her cycle to give a blood sample for these tests. The doctor prefers day two because, in her opinion, tests conducted on this day provide the most accurate output and gives her the feasibility she needs to be able to offer her patients the best care and treatment derived from their unique circumstances. She believes running these tests outside this window would be like taking a snapshot of a moving object where you end up with a blurry or an inaccurate output.

Cycle day two finally arrives for Christina. They run the tests, and the results show that Christina's hormones are imbalanced, which explains why she's been having difficulties conceiving. She will have to be put on medications to get this issue resolved.

Comparing the two scenarios between doctor one and doctor two, Christina feels like she is finally getting somewhere. Doctor one shows little to no signs of professionalism and compassion. She is very quick to send Christina home without trying to analyze her situation. Doctor two, on the other hand, demonstrates a high level of professionalism, is full of compassion, and is very solution oriented. Why would Christina not choose doctor two over doctor one? At this point, she can safely say she has found a good doctor she can trust to handle her case, and she is extremely delighted about that.

CHAPTER 11

Lessons Learned

Phase 1 of this book details Christina's journey with her attempt to start a family. But before we dive into that, let's benefit from some of the lessons she has learned so far as she speaks to us in this chapter.

My loss had taken total control of me. It was so bad that I became insane with long intervals of horrible sanity. It is completely sane to be sad and cry over a loss, but being sad or crying about it repeatedly will not erase the loss. Learning how to live with it is far better than immersing yourself in circles of sadness and expecting some sort of healing to magically occur.

Believe me when I tell you that I cried buckets and buckets of tears when I experienced my loss in August 2014. As a matter of fact, it had become a habit for me to curl up in my bed or on my couch and cry all day, longing for the pain to go away.

Nothing in the world had any meaning to me anymore. Slowly but surely, I closed myself off from everyone and everything around me to my own detriment. The sad truth is that adopting this way of life did not take the pain away, and it didn't bring my baby back. If anything, I rather became insane in my sanity. I had to make a conscious effort to change my ways in order to get different results or crash and burn in my misery.

I am glad I took the leap of faith and brawled my way back to sanity, for it is through the brawling that I learned a tremendous number of lessons that have contributed enormously in making me a better person today. My journey brought me to the realization that life is truly a succession of lessons that must be lived to be understood. Of all the many lessons learned from my situation, I have chosen my top seven (in no particular order of importance) to share with you.

Lesson 1: Support Your Spouse

No one seems to realize that Tim is equally in pain. The pain of losing his baby and seeing how much pain I am experiencing on a daily basis is cutting deeply right through his chest and into his heart. A world that was once so bright has suddenly gone dim, crashing around him right before his own eyes. But like most men will do, Tim feels obliged to keep it together and be strong for the family, especially for me, comforting me through it all, always holding me, and wiping my tears away as they drop. He goes through his day doing what he is supposed to do as the head of our household even with a heart that has been ripped apart abruptly like a cheap piece of fabric. He constantly hides behind a mask when he is feeling melancholy, bottling up his fears and smiling through his tears.

But what people are seeing on the outside is not real. It is the complete opposite of what this gentle man is actually going through. He puts up this stout image, but deep inside, his heart is broken, and he is as weak as a vegetable. Like most men, Tim doesn't always show how he truly feels. He conceals his feelings and emotions, and when he is alone, that's when the tears start flowing like water from a broken pipe. He searches for answers but can't find any. He hurts. He hurts so badly. His son he so wanted to meet is gone like the wind.

Forthrightly speaking, we are receiving tremendous support from family and friends, but most of it is geared toward me, Christina. All flowers and cards are addressed to me. When phone calls come in, they are looking to speak with me. Almost everyone will ask Tim how I am doing but will hardly remember to ask him how he is coping with the loss. It's all about Christina and little to nothing about Tim.

The terrible truth at the kernel of losing a child is that we as human beings (men and women alike) find it almost impossible to make sense of it. It goes against every grain in our psyche. It's not the natural order of things, and we know the world was not meant to be that way, so we hurt. The grieving mom hurts, and so does the grieving dad. It is a horrifying loss for both parents and not just the woman.

Sadly, whenever such a tragedy strikes, most people tend to sympathize more with the mother, and I guess that's probably because she carried the baby in her womb. They forget about the father who is also suffering an incredible loss. Although he didn't carry the baby, his loss is equally true and deep. He just lost his child, for crying out loud. All his dreams, hopes, and expectations for that baby have been shattered. However, society somehow forgets that he is hurting. Rather, they expect and throw so much at him during this delicate moment.

Let's take my situation as an example here. I couldn't have done it without my amazing husband. He went above and beyond for me when we experienced the most traumatic thing life has ever thrown at us. With me having a roller coaster of emotions after the loss, I can assure you that I wasn't a very pleasant person to be around most of the time. I was dealing with a lot of confusing emotions ranging from disbelief to a lot of anger, guilt, and sadness in my life—more than I've ever thought possible. But through it all, my husband was there for me in every way imaginable, and that made the grieving process a little less difficult, or at least a whole lot easier to acknowledge and accept what I was going through.

Dejectedly, I didn't realize how much effort he was putting in just to make sure I got the support I needed because I was busy expecting. Yeah! I was expecting him to be a superman, forgetting that he himself was grieving and in need of emotional and psychological support as well. I wasn't different from society. I was throwing too much at my husband even when he was trying so hard through his pain to be there for me, comforting and supporting me the best he could.

Just like society, I had made the situation about me and not about us. I had gradually replaced the all-powerful *we* in a relationship with *I*, slowly turning our partnership into a sole proprietorship without realizing it. I had become so incredibly selfish and distasteful. I rarely appreciated anything he did during that period because I felt entitled to it. How he managed to keep his composure during these trying times is something I've still been unable to fully comprehend and probably never will.

Coming to the realization that I had not given enough thought and consideration to how my husband was feeling about our loss brought a lot of shame on me. It cut me so deep. I sobbed for days and still do occasionally whenever those horrible feelings of guilt creep in. I've tendered countless apologies for being so selfish, but I still feel like it's not enough. The good thing is that he has forgiven me. He forgave me even before I realized the awful person my emotions had turned me into.

Thinking a little deeper, this man was literally in a deep, dark valley but still found ways to do the most amazing things just to see a smile on my face. He did everything within his capacity under the sun to make sure I was happy even when I failed to appreciate him. He never wavered. He remained very consistent and stayed true to himself, uplifting the value of those marriage vows we made that read, "I, Tim, take you Christina as my lawful wedded wife, to have and to hold, from this day forward, for better or worse, for richer or poorer, in sickness and in health, until death do us part." How incredible!

I don't know about your exact situation, but I can only speak from my own life experiences, hoping they can in some way help you handle yours better if such a tragedy were to befall you. Keep in mind that when a couple grows together, it becomes inevitable that they will see each other through life's most tumultuous and traumatic experiences, including, but not limited to, illness, loss, failure, death, and so on. No matter what the case may be, always remember that dads and men in general hurt, grieve, and need support.

We as human beings are different. Our struggles with difficult situations are unique and individual to each and every one of us. We grieve differently, and there is no right or wrong way to grieve. We cannot expect our partners to be mirror images of ourselves. Rather, we should remember that we are our partner's safe place and give them the room and the freedom to grieve in their own personal and unique way that works for them. We as individuals vary enormously in how we experience grief, including its intensity, its duration, and even how we express it.

Moreover, men do not grieve in the same exact way as women. Women tend to express their feelings and even seek support from others, while men tend to internalize their feelings and deal with loss on their own. They often feel the need to take care of their partners by remaining strong for them during unfortunate moments. It is not uncommon to misread your partner's stoicism as not caring about you and/or your loss if you don't understand this behavior.

Bereavement is a very complex, dynamic, and fragile process that does not necessarily proceed in any orderly linear fashion. We rather all have concurrent and overlapping reactions that may actually recur at any time during the grieving process. We cannot assume that we know exactly how the other is feeling and pass judgment. But what we can do is this: be there for them, listen to them, hold them, run errands for them, sit in silence with them, take them out for a meal, go for a walk with them, plan recreational activities for them, and so on and so forth.

If anything, our partners are always the first persons we turn to in difficult times. Even if society doesn't realize that your husband/partner is in deep grief, it is our responsibility as spouses to remember and make a conscious effort to support them. It is important that your partner knows that you are there for him during a tragic moment. Ladies/moms, we aren't the only ones that hurt; dads/men hurt too.

Lesson 2: Society's Expectations and Reactions

When we experienced our loss, people reacted to us in a variety of ways. There were some who genuinely condoned with us and supported us in every way possible, some who expected us to behave in a certain way, others who sobbed whenever they called us or saw us, and others who never asked what happened to the growing belly.

The love, care, and concern we received during our grief was enormous. There were people who stopped by the hospital every evening on their way back from work just to see how we were doing. Others came with flowers and others with food. Some prayed for us and with us. We had some who were far away and called multiple times a day to check on us. Even when we went home, the trend continued. We were never alone. We were surrounded by a lot of love and support from family, friends, and well-wishers, and we remain grateful to them for all the sacrifices they made and continue to make to be there for us.

Credit to my good friend Elaine who flew in all the way from Atlanta just to be by my side during the tragedy. This is something I really appreciate and something that I will forever be grateful for. She was so introspective, and I do not take it for granted. When she got the news regarding my situation, she rushed to her computer and purchased a last-minute plane ticket with the speed of light. When she arrived the airport, she was informed that her ticket had been booked to depart from Baltimore/Washington International (BWI) Airport to Hartsfield-Jackson Atlanta International Airport and not the other way around as she believed. Poor thing!

Luckily, there was an outbound flight to Baltimore scheduled for departure within the next couple of hours, and the airlines managed to reverse the booking, although it came at an additional cost to her as you would imagine. While on the plane, the flight attendants on behalf of the airlines, made a very nice gesture by offering her a beautiful teddy bear with a get-well-soon note to bring to me, which I still have to date. That was so thoughtful and kind of them to do. She arrived in Baltimore right before midnight and made it to my hospital room by 1:30 a.m. I was delighted to see her. Elaine stayed with me for a few days before flying back home.

On the other hand of the spectrum, some people or societal expectations didn't make it easy on us during this difficult moment. Ideally, grieving parents should have the right to behave exactly as their instincts direct them. I should be able to cry whenever I want to for as long as I want and as loud as I want or not cry at all. I should be able to get angry if I want to, smile or laugh if I want to, groom myself in whatever way I want, or not groom myself if I don't feel like it. Whatever I do should be entirely up to me. After all, isn't mourning supposed to be an individual's unique process of adaptation following the loss of a loved one?

Unfortunately, it's not always the case in the world we live in. The irony is that while society acknowledged the scale and intensity of our loss, it proceeded to erect a very strict frame of reference regarding what is deemed as acceptable behavior following a loss. There are all sorts of unwritten, socially prescribed methods of how we are supposed to respond to a loss, including, but not limited to, our external expressions and behaviors such as rituals and memorials.

In my case, I was considered as being too engulfed in my grief. People constantly talked me out of expressing my pain the way my instincts were directing me. Rather than doing what felt right for me, I found myself trying to fit into this invisible narrow frame of what was expected of me. I was constantly fighting and holding back tears because people felt that I was crying too much. Sometimes I hide under my sheets and cry for fear of being judged.

Instead of me dealing with my grief as it surfaced, I was trying to pressure myself to get past the pain quickly because that's what society expects of me. They expect me to grieve for a certain amount of time and then magically expunge everything and move on to doing bigger and greater things. I can tell you right now that this method didn't cut the chase for me. Grief is a process that must be completed in order to experience healing, and I find healing to be more complete if you deal with your grief as it comes. Pressure to heal and bounce back just doesn't gel together with grief. Your emotions need time to recover, so take your time to heal.

A friend visited with me on my fourth day in the hospital following the incident and told me to my face that I wasn't crying enough. While I was trying to be strong on the outside and doing what society expected of me, my own friend expected me to be very gloomy and on the verge of tears. Isn't it confusing when you factor in the bunch that considered me to be too engulfed in my grief? Here is what she said to me with a rising intonation: "Are you sure you just lost a baby? I can't believe you aren't even crying. If I were you, I would have died by now. I can't imagine anything happening to any of my kids."

It took every ounce of patience in me to not punch her in the face, and I mean every single word of what I just said. I wanted to smash her in the face. How dare she? To some, you are crying more than you should, while others think you are not crying enough, and both voices are so insistent. I was lost trying to respond to people's expectations instead of working through my feelings on my own terms. There were even some people who completely avoided any conversation about the loss, often uttering dismissing statements such as the following.

"It is better he passed away when you hadn't met him and established a bond."

"You are still young and can always have another child."

"God needed another flower in his garden."

"I know exactly how you feel."

"At least you know that you can get pregnant. Some people can't. Just try again."

"Everything happens for a reason."

"It's been too long now. You have to let it go in order to create space for the next baby."

How rude! These are not very helpful things to say to a grieving mother or father. They are completely off the mark and distressing. Words are powerful and can have long-lasting effects either positively or negatively on how a person feels, acts, and reacts. Use words that will uplift and not dampen. Use words of affirmation, affinity, love, and care. We can do better, and we should strive to do better.

In retrospect, while I don't fault these individuals for saying such things because I believe their messages and words were very well-intentioned, I must admit that those messages and words are exceedingly painful. It almost feels like they disregard your loss or that your baby's demise means nothing to them. It leaves you worse off than you were before they approached you with such dismissal consolations.

I remember being apprehensive around people who used one or a combination of the above-mentioned painful phrases in an effort to provide support when we encountered our loss. I didn't feel comfortable engaging in conversations with them, and I did everything within my power to avoid any avenue that could lead to such; I screened calls, changed topics of conversation, intentionally stayed away from gatherings where I suspected they would be, and so much more. I just did not want to deal with them because I found them toxic.

On the other hand, I was drawn to those who provided a safe, nonjudgmental space for me to grieve. These people would ask me how I was doing, how I was feeling, and if there was anything they could do to make me feel better. They actively listened to me and provided beautiful messages of affirmation, affinity, love, and care. They reassured me that it wasn't my fault whenever I tried to blame myself for the event. They were there for me, and I could feel it deep within my soul, and that was very sweet of them.

Lesson 3: Self-forgiveness

Learning to forgive yourself is vital part in this process. I was dealing with a lot of unforgiveness in my life after our loss. I kept asking myself if there was something I did or something I failed to do that led to the events of August 4, 2014. I wrestled with my thoughts day and night, trying to find answers to no avail. I would look at my medical reports and get even more frustrated by the fact that every single thing appeared normal. I was constantly off-balance and blamed myself for the loss of our baby. Deep within, I believed there was something I could have done to make him stay.

I could never wrap my head around what exactly I should have or could have done to prevent the circumstances from occurring. The poison of unforgiveness was eating me up and killing me slowly. No matter how hard I tried to heal, it wasn't really happening. I was trapped by the monster called unforgiveness for a significant amount of time. When I started accepting the fact that the abruption didn't happen because of me, but rather, it happened to me, I started embracing the willingness to forgive myself.

To date, this remains one of the best decisions I've ever made. I experienced such a great moment of liberation when I decided to forgive myself, let go of the burden, and walk into a new path of promise and hope for the future. Forgiveness is undoubtedly one of the most precious gifts you can ever gift yourself. It opens the door to change by releasing resistance and deepening the connection you have/feel toward yourself.

The ability to forgive yourself is critical to your psychological well-being. Forgive yourself, think kind thoughts toward yourself, and show yourself some compassion. You deserve it. Forgiving what we cannot forget creates a new way to remember. We change the memory of our past into a hope for the future by forgiving ourselves.

Lesson 4: The Past

Unfortunately, once the past is done, we cannot go back and undo it. Holding on to a past event that has negative connotations will not help you. If anything, it rather has the potential to imprison you and destroy your future. As harsh as it may sound, let the past stay in the past where it belongs. Stop hauling it around. Once I got to the point where I was able to truly acknowledge that our baby's passing was now an event that occurred in the past and couldn't be undone, I started opening myself to more acceptance. The more I accepted the fact that our little boy was gone for good, the better I felt.

Increased acceptance is not easy, but it is such a powerful step and has been an enormous contributing factor in our emotional healing process. Emotional healing does not happen overnight. It is a process that requires time and patience. It is not the same for everyone. But no matter how long it takes, there is light at the end of the tunnel. Do not give up in the process, for there is hope, and I can testify to that because I have lived it.

Losing a baby is one of the most painful things that can happen to a parent or family in general. Some may snap out of it easily, and some may never really get over it. There is no right amount of time to get over this process, and it's also okay to never get over it at all. Let it take as long as it takes for you.

I won't say that I've gotten over the loss of our baby and left it in the past where it belongs; however, I can safely say that I have moved through my grief to a place of healing, and part of it is largely due to increased acceptance that our baby is gone. I have created a special place in my heart and mind for the memories of my baby. My husband and I often remember how excited the baby would get whenever we watched a soccer game, be it in person or on television. We remember how he moved around in my belly and respond to our inside jokes. We have lots of fun memories of our baby boy that will live with us forever.

With time, we've found peace, and we hope that over time, you can find peace too and become ready to think about what the future holds.

Lesson 5: Open Up

Opening up about your loss, grief, and pain helps tremendously, but I understand that it can be a very hard thing to do. In general terms, we are not brought up being trained on how to process loss and pain or on how to openly talk about such feelings. Looking at it keenly, it can be very uncomfortable on two fronts.

On one front, the person experiencing the pain might shy away from talking about it because he or she fears coming across as weak. On the other front, the listener finds it painful to see a loved one in pain. Somehow, mirror neurons in our brains do make us feel our loved ones' pain as if it were ours.

In addition, human beings are not wired to find pleasure in pain, so people might withdraw and avoid listening to anything that might make them feel bad. Most people hardly know how to react or what to say in such circumstances except for the golden safe words: "I'm so sorry."

In my case, when some people tried to go beyond how sorry they felt for me when I suffered my loss, most of them inadvertently said things like: "Whether baby is gone or not, life goes on, and you should too." "You've been mourning for too long. You can't keep doing this to yourself. Get over it." Although they said it with good intentions, these things hurt rather than help. Today with my renewed mature mind, I don't fault them because they are not trained to deal with such issues.

No matter how awful someone or people may have made you feel in the past in the process of you trying to express your feelings, do not give up. It is very unhealthy to suppress your feelings. The pain you are experiencing is emotional and psychological and cannot be overlooked. As a matter of fact, suppressing your feelings is an important public health concern.

Losing my baby to unexpected death came with a lot of excruciating pain—pain that is worse than physical pain simply because no one can see it, leaving people with the assumption that you are fine when in actuality you are bleeding on the inside and feel like dying. When you are experiencing grief, you are everything but fine. There is this deep inside injury you've sustained, which I call a psychological wound. This wound can be likened to a physical wound except for the fact that a physical wound is visible, and a psychological wound is invisible. Both are excruciatingly painful and take time and proper care to heal.

Metaphorically speaking, there are similarities in the healing process of both wounds. If you've ever had a wound, you may remember that the first step a health professional took was to make sure they cleaned your wound before applying any form of medicine to it. If physical wounds are not cleaned and treated, they will get infected and pose an even greater threat. The same logic applies to emotional and psychological wounds. They must be cleaned first. In its healing process, the cleaning is done by talking about it and letting feelings our out.

A major step in working through this kind of pain is allowing yourself to be vulnerable about your struggles. The more you talk or write about it, the easier it gets, but the more you try to suppress it, the more likely your invisible wound will get infected, leaving you with more bitter struggles. Pain will not disappear if you suppress it, and unresolved issues will not be resolved if you refuse to accept them and talk about them.

I found out that when I started writing and talking about my inner wounds, the pain began subsiding and becoming more bearable. As social creatures, not only do we feel better when we open up about our struggles, but we help others in similar situations to find ways of dealing with their challenges. To me, this has been one of my greatest accomplishments. Seeing someone being motivated by my story is very heartwarming, humbling, and rewarding. You can't afford to burry your pain and miss out on the goodness that comes with opening yourself up. If anything, it builds you; it doesn't burn you.

There are many steps that you can take as you go through this process. You can find someone you resonate with and feel safe and comfortable with to talk to. You can join a support group in your community where you can meet and open up to people who are going through similar experiences. You will be amazed at how listening to other stories of loss and healing from unexpected people allows you to feel less alone and helps you heal.

You may be crushed or even feel numb and surrounded by family and friends who may not understand, and that's okay. Find someone who does. Finding understanding and support from unexpected people can also give you some clarity into why some of the people you expect to understand you don't seem to get how much you are hurting. They've never been there, which makes it hard for them to know what it's like. Some people truly mean well and want to say something comforting but just don't know what exactly to say. Try not to take it personally if they say the wrong thing or nothing at all.

You could also seek professional help to help you grapple with the difficult emotions you are experiencing and ultimately come to terms with your grief. This could be from anyone who is qualified and specialized in helping people cope with such issues. It could be a therapist, psychologists, life coach, or priest. I strongly encourage you to open up, my dear friends.

Together, let's experience freedom and enjoy the golden opportunity to inspire others given our unique experiences.

To those of you who just can't break that shell you are in or who cannot pull down that invisible wall you've built in order to hide your pain, I urge you to reflect on the following words: Stagnant water breeds mosquitoes and forms algae and eventually diseases. However, if there is a controlled flow of water from the source into a crater and out of the crater to other parts of its surroundings, the water in the crater stays clean, maintains life downstream, and leaves plenty of clean water in the crater. Which would you rather be: stagnant water or water in the crater from a controlled source? I really wish and hope you choose the latter.

Lesson 6: Dealing with Dark and Bad Days

Taking my tragedy into consideration, you know I've had to deal with a lot of dark days. As a matter of fact, we've all had to deal with dark days at some point in our lives, and we are bound to have them again. Bad days interchange like the weather except for the absence of forecasted predictability or patterns. They can be terrible and terrifying, but one thing I learned from dealing with dark days is this: They won't make you feel better. Rather, they will drain you and destroy you.

The fact that we are having a bad day doesn't mean we are having a bad life. It doesn't even mean the world has come to an end. Life continues after a bad day. No matter how dark the clouds may appear, there is always light between them. The sun is still in existence, and there is always tomorrow, which could be much brighter than today. This realization switched my outlook and changed my life completely for the better. I made a conscious decision to change the way I think and start handling my bad days differently.

I will no longer pave the way for negativity and mediocrity. It had become a habit for me to get all gloomy and grumpy and curl up and cry in a hidden corner whenever I felt a bit melancholy. This didn't help the situation. If anything, I was trapped in the whirlwind of my own thoughts with no purpose. I am grateful that in that dark place, I was able to find ways of tackling bad days better whenever they occur. The obstacles of one's past can truly become gateways that will eventually lead to new beginnings. Below are some of the strategies that helped me get back up.

Express Gratitude for What You Already Have:

Bad days should not erase the good things we've done or the good we've gotten out of this life. Each time I encounter a bad day, I try to direct my focus on the positives in my life by visualizing the things I've been blessed with (life, health, spouse, family, friends, accomplishments, etc.) and express profound gratitude for them. When I'm done being grateful, I come to the realization that I had no reason to be breaking down in the first place. Instead, there is so much to be grateful for. Why break down?

This strategy helped me so much during my healing process, and today, it has become a daily routine for me. Just by setting aside ten to thirty seconds each day to express gratitude for the things I have, my overall well-being has increased remarkably. Ten to thirty seconds of reflection and gratitude actually help the brain to rewire itself commit that positive moment into a memory. It tends to be the shake-up my brain needs to jump-start my day with positive energy. It's amazing how focusing on the positives can change the way you think.

Train yourself to switch your thoughts, and you will not regret your effort. Whenever those bad blues come creeping in, they come with a lot of pressure. Try not to put any additional pressure on yourself. Instead, try to think of something that has brought you enormous joy in the past, and soak yourself in those memories. If I had to assume, I would say there must be at least one memory from everyone's past that is filled with beautiful emotions. Recalling that special memory and the connection you made at the time can make you feel better.

Exercise

The benefits of exercise cannot be overemphasized, my dear friends. Did you know that exercise helps release serotonin receptors in the brain, a chemical responsible for maintaining mood balance? Research shows that a deficit of serotonin leads to depression. The more you exercise, the more receptors your brain produces, and the better your mood is. Exercise is like a reset button, and it only takes about twenty minutes to get its full mental and physical benefits. Setting aside about a half hour each day to exercise will go a long way to help you not only during bad days but will equally increase your overall well-being.

Stepping out of the house and exercising outside was particularly helpful for me because I admire and appreciate nature so much. When I'm outside taking a walk, seeing the beauty of nature, its variability, and all the sounds and smells sort of shifts my brain and body into a very positive mental state. I become very relaxed and happy and always end up walking longer than the distance I originally set out for.

Be mindful of the fact that doing the same exercise over and over can easily become boring or demotivate you, and this is the last thing you want in this process. There is a plethora of things you can incorporate into your routine in order to stay in check. Find a variety of activities you enjoy doing. It can also be helpful to join a group of people who enjoy the same activities as you. Meetup is a great platform for this. I've met the most incredible people through meetup groups. Find a workout buddy or a coach or trainer who can motivate you and keep you accountable. Set exercise goals for yourself, start slow, and work your way up to meet your target.

The moral here is that unhappiness and despair soak up a lot of energy. In fact, any emotion takes energy, but unhappiness often feels like very hard physical labor. Rather than being unhappy and wearing yourself out on unproductive situations, I encourage you to make the choice to take that same energy and harness its power for better things that you can be proud of. Divert your energy away from unhappiness and channel it toward a more useful purpose.

Set goals for yourself and learn how to use the momentum and energy that you have within to accelerate the process of achieving those goals. This can be a challenging but also very rewarding process. Taking that very first step is always a challenge in most circumstances and often requires some ingenuity. Remember that connecting your energy to a purpose can take many different forms.

In my case, for example, I came to the realization that focusing on my hobbies gives me the motivation to pull myself out of unhappy moods.

Doing the things you love can be incredibly meditative and helpful in converting negative energy into positive energy. Find what works for you and stick to it.

Lesson 7: Attitude

The only good factor I can think of to get the lesson I learned about attitude across is to mention my motivation: Prince Harry. My write-up on what helped me to come forward with my struggles is stirred by Prince Harry's candid admission to his struggles with mental health in an extraordinary podcast interview with Bryony Gordon in April 2017. His story clearly illustrates the fact that attitude is an inward feeling expressed by outward behavior hinged on past experiences. Its roots are inward, but its fruit is outward. It can be seen or noticed without a word being altered, and it is more honest and more consistent than our words.

Note that of all the things we wear, our expression is the most important and most remembered. Prior to identifying and tackling the underlying cause of his issues, the prince's past attitude dictated undesirable results not only to him but also to his family and friends. A hardened attitude is a dreaded disease that causes a closed mind and a dark future. It wasn't until he paused, examined himself, and took action that things started to change for him in a positive direction. When attitude becomes positive and conducive for growth, the mind expands, progress begins, and outward expressions become desirable.

One thing I've come to realize about attitude is that it can be formed, learned, changed, and/or reinforced at any point in our lives. There is no such thing as an unalterable attitude. Whatever bad attitudes you have adopted can be altered to work in your favor. As a matter of fact, our attitudes do need some remodeling or adjustments with every change that comes into our lives. We all will encounter storms at some point in our lives that will threaten to wreck the healthy attitudes we've built over the years.

When tragedy hits, it is natural to bail out of the right attitude to compensate for our problems. We tend to internalize our unfortunate circumstances instead of trying to make a conscious effort to adopt a rewarding positive attitude. When we internalize our unfortunate external difficulties, they lead to wrong internal reactions, and that's when the difficulty really becomes a problem. Our internal reactions begin to surface on the outside through our unpleasant actions.

In my case, not only had I suffered an unexpected placental abruption that led to the loss of my baby and a miserable life, but I also started having problems getting pregnant. I was completely lost and gradually turning from a bubbly, pleasant individual with a positive outlook on life to an odious, negative, unpleasant person with a very negative outlook on life. Slowly but surely, I shifted from being an extroverted person to becoming an introvert, and whenever I spoke, nothing good came out. I communicated less with family and friends. I even became a not-so-pleasant wife.

Prior to my unfortunate circumstances, my husband was my knight in shining armor. We illustrated beautiful ideas and worked incredibly well together. We built on each other's strengths and expected the best from ourselves. I ignored anything that seemed to be a weakness in him. I saw him as a man with noble feelings and fine qualities. Our marriage was fun, and we enjoyed doing life together.

Things changed dramatically after the loss and the struggle. I became horrendous. I ignored all his strengths and focused on his weaknesses. I stopped encouraging him on his endeavors and began expecting the worst. We stopped working well together. Our once beautiful relationship had taken a sharp, stiff turn downhill. Do you see how damaging an unhealthy attitude can be? Is it really what you want? I don't think so. Make it a habit to work on your attitude whenever you are faced with uncomfortable situations. It worked and continues to work for me, and I believe it can work for you too.

Words of Encouragement

Although any death of a loved one can be emotionally devastating, population-based studies in the United States show that unexpected deaths provoke especially strong responses, as there is less time to prepare for and adapt to the circumstances. If you've experienced any kind of loss, know that your emotions are valid.

I understand how profound, difficult, and painful it is to experience infant loss because I have lived it. I know about the difficulty in believing that you've actually lost your baby, the feeling that life is empty, the feeling that a part of you has died, the feeling that your world has been shattered, the feeling of worthlessness, the irritability, the extreme levels of bitterness, the feeling of anger, the inability to concentrate, the confusion, the frustration, the sadness, the despair, the anxiety, the panic attacks, the loss of appetite, the insomnia, the obsessive thinking, and so on that come with grief. I've lived them all, and I'm here to encourage you to believe that there is hope after a loss because there truly is hope.

Our loss was unthinkable, unanticipated, and horrifying, and that literally took us to a very low, dark, cold place—a place we've never envisioned to exist even in our wildest imaginations, and a place surrounded by loneliness, misery, and hopelessness with no purpose for the future. It literally hits you like a strong wave of mass destruction, and you get this profound feeling of instability. It feels like the earth isn't stable anymore. Trust me when I tell you that I know how it feels because I do.

Months, weeks, days, and even the morning of the day of the unfortunate tragedy were all filled with so much peace, joy, and happiness in our lives. Life felt fabulous. But while I was soaking under the radiance of the sun, I had no clue that invisible black clouds were looming above me, ready to pour by the afternoon. Oh! August 4, 2014 … What a day! A day that started out so bright, sunny, and lovely ended with an unexpected tornado that flipped my world in the complete opposite direction of where I was headed. Our precious, adorable little boy left us without an opportunity to just open his eyes to see the outside world even for a second. Not even a chance to cry his first cry. How cruel! How cruel! How do I pick up my pieces and move on? Can I even move on? I asked myself all these questions and more in my pain and misery.

Thankfully, we were able to find something solid beneath our feet that contributed tremendously in helping us climb back out of rock bottom. I am more than pleased and excited to share with you some of the things that gave us strength during our struggle, hoping that you can be encouraged in one way or the other.

1. Maintain the right attitude.

In order to stay sane and secure a safe landing, I had to learn to continually adjust and stretch my attitude through the raging storm. I can now safely say that just by changing my attitude, I transformed a miserable situation into a highly rewarding one. Being a travel lover, I started traveling more. I've been to the most amazing dreamlike places around the world, and I've learned so much about different cultures and cuisines in the last few years.

I've also experienced many different adventures that I never imagined possible. Things such as underwater walking, paragliding, bungee jumping, elephant trekking, skydiving, and so on are things I never envisioned myself doing. Today, I can proudly say they've been checked off my bucket list. When your attitude is right, not only does the future look bright, but the present also becomes more enjoyable. Your attitude truly determines your approach to life.

Think about this seriously. I had the choice to either continue to be caught up in my pain, capitalize on it, and remain miserable or to stretch my attitude, free myself from that prison, and enjoy life. I'm so glad I went with the more rewarding choice, and I strongly encourage you to do the same. Do not let your misery shrink your life. Let it stretch you. I no longer view my adversities as the sunset of life. I view them as the sunrise of a bright new opportunity. Did you know that every difficulty presents an opportunity and every opportunity presents a difficulty?

To further illustrate this, permit me to liken adversities to a grindstone. It can either grind you down or polish you up depending on what you are made of or the kind of attitude you adopt. Remember the quote by Lou Holtz that reads: "Life is 10% what happens to you and 90% how you respond to it"? The importance of attitude cannot be overemphasized. It is the one string we have when life happens to us. Our attitude is the single-most important thing when we encounter tough times. In order words, how we respond to our crisis can either make us or break us from that point forward.

Let's look at some of my favorite strong, influential individuals who encountered tough times but turned their tragedies into positives by maintaining a positive attitude toward life.

Helen Adams Keller

The deaf and blind author, political activist, and lecturer definitely knew what she was talking about when she said, "Although the world is full of suffering, it is also full of overcoming it." Born with her senses of sight and hearing, Helen started speaking when she was just six months old. Despondently, at nineteen months old, she contracted a rare disease that left her deaf and blind. She toiled for years to learn to speak and mastered several methods of communication just so she could be able to communicate and be understood by others. She didn't give up. At the age of twenty-four, she graduated college and became a social activist. During her lifetime, she received many honors in recognition of her accomplishments, including the Theodore Roosevelt Distinguished Service Medal in 1936 and the Presidential Medal of Freedom in 1964. She was elected to the Women's Hall of Fame in 1965. She also received honorary doctoral degrees from Temple University, Harvard University, and other universities around the globe, including Glasgow, Scotland; Berlin, Germany; India; and Witwatersrand in Johannesburg, South Africa. Helen died in 1968 just before her eighty-eighth birthday. What a remarkable life and a stunning example of how hard work and determination can turn things around for your good.

She overcame the adversity of being deaf and blind and became one of the twentieth century's leading humanitarians. No matter how colossal your adversities may appear, you have the ability in you to triumph over them. Helen had every reason to give up on life, but she didn't. To her, self-pity was unacceptable, and failure was not an option. That's the kind of attitude you need to adopt. If stories as such do not encourage you to adopt a positive outlook and keep moving, then I don't know what will.

Emilie Gossiaux

As a little girl growing up in Louisiana, Emilie could see, but she was deaf at just five years of age and needed a hearing aid in each ear to help her with her disability. She loved art and had a great determination to become an artist. She spent most of her time making sketches. In 2007, she was admitted into Manhattan's Cooper Union School of Art. Life was great, and Emilie was living her dreams until the morning of Friday October 8, 2010, when an eighteen-wheeler truck, upon taking a turn at the corner of Johnson and Varick in Brooklyn, New York, plowed right over the twenty-one-year-old, crushing her severely.

She suffered a traumatic brain injury, stroke, multiple lacerations all over her body, and fractures to her head, pelvis, and legs. The accident also left her blind. While at the hospital, doctors worked frantically to save her life and saw no hope. They didn't believe she would recover and didn't think she was a candidate for rehabilitation. Her situation was so bad that nurses were asking her parents if they wanted to donate her organs.

Although the health care team saw a vegetable when they looked at Emilie, her parents and her boyfriend saw a fighter. They refused to accept the prognosis and didn't give up hope. They did everything within their power to help Emilie, and slowly but surely, she began responding. Eventually, she was able to start talking again, but that was just the beginning of the fight, as she still had to learn how to communicate and how to do everything all over again.

Faced with this tragedy and now being blind brought another limitation and difficulty to Emilie, but amazingly, she didn't give up. She was rather more determined and hungrier for success than ever before. She didn't let her disabilities limit her. She found ways of overcoming them in order to achieve her dream of becoming an artist. She learned braille (a tactile reading and writing system used by people who are visually impaired). On average, it takes two years to learn braille, but due to the burning desire in Emilie to succeed, she learned this tactile system and finished reading her first braille book all within a year.

In the spring of 2013, she went back to Cooper Union to complete her undergraduate degree. A few months down the road, she won an Award of Excellence from the Kennedy Center for Performing Arts for a stunning sculpture (*Bird Sitting*) she had created two years after her accident. A year later, she graduated college, and today she continues to create art that inspires people across the globe.

Oprah Winfrey

Although Oprah is one of the most successful women in the world today, she too had to work through some very deep adversities to develop into who she is today. Born into poverty in rural Mississippi, being sexually abused at a tender age of nine, falling pregnant at fourteen, and losing her baby just after giving birth were enough to throw her off the wagon, but it didn't. Why? Because she remained strong and didn't let her circumstances take control of her. She continued school and even became an honors student in high school, which earned her a full scholarship for college.

She graduated college and was turned down when she interviewed for jobs, but that still didn't stop Oprah. She kept pressing on and ended up hosting her own talk show and even became one of the most powerful and influential women in the world. In 1995, she featured on *Forbes* 400 list of richest Americans. In 2005, she ranked ninth on the *Forbes* Top 10 Most Powerful Women in the World list and third in 2010. Today, she owns a multibillion-dollar fortune, and *Forbes* lists her as one of America's richest self-made women. If she had given up, none of the above would have been realized. She is truly a force to reckon with.

What is common with the abovementioned icons is not only the fact that they've all been through some excruciating times in their lives but also that in those tough times they all recognized that a struggle is a stepping-stone to what lies ahead. They were all able to overcome their adversities and turn them into positives. Whenever I think about these three stout women, I am reminded of the fact that no matter what I've been through in life or may be going through, it is not over. If you are willing to do whatever it takes to turn things around in your favor, stick to it, and maintain the right attitude, you can rebound. Your comeback story is ready to be written—but only when you are ready to fully commit. When darkness shows up in your life, the right attitude to maintain is not to curse the darkness but rather to light a candle. The lit candle will bring light and help you see clearly to maneuver your way out of the dark. It is better to light a candle than to curse the darkness.

PHASE 2

Fertility Struggles and Its Consequences

(Inspired by My Unique Experience)

INTRODUCTION

One of the most common misconceptions of having a family is the belief that we will be able to have children once we are ready to do so. This assumption is not challenged until a couple encounters difficulties in the process of trying to conceive. The path to parenthood is less than straightforward for some women, including myself and many others. Although our journeys with fertility struggles are not identical, most of our experiences are connected.

It is emotionally, physically, and financially exhausting. It completely consumes your body and your life like a raging, odious monster, and it makes you forget who you are. You literally begin living your life one month at a time, hoping for a positive pregnancy test every single cycle as you navigate a very tight schedule of appointments, tests, and treatments. While going through this, you also have to watch your family members, friends, and even coworkers become mothers, sometimes more than once, and you have to be happy for them and sad for yourself at the same time. That's what I call a sophisticated endurance test—look happy when you feel hollow and sad.

Unfortunately, the conversation about fertility struggles still carries a stigma. The lack of empathy toward individuals struggling with their fertility results in many people keeping a stiff upper lip about these grueling scuffles, creating a misunderstanding about what it's truly like when embroiled in it.

CHAPTER 1

My Fertility Journey

To encapsulate phase 1 of my story, I went from getting pregnant without trying to losing my baby at a very advanced stage in my pregnancy and later on finding myself on the fertility struggle bus, fighting tooth and nail to achieve another pregnancy. This all happened too quickly and scarred me in so many areas. It was and still feels like a cruel twist of fate that's more than enough to break a human being, but through all of this, I realize how blessed I am to have the opportunity to not only be alive after facing a near-death situation but also to be able to benefit from assisted reproductive technologies (ARTs) in my battle with fertility.

Although nerve-wracking and confusing, it all started with a pretty straightforward process where my doctor gave me a detailed explanation of my test results, emphasizing on the numbers, what they meant, and possible ways forward in my quest for a baby. After struggling for years with medicated cycles in an attempt to fall pregnant, in vitro fertilization (IVF) sounded like the ultimate choice to go for at this point. I was diagnosed with unexplained infertility and told that based off of my numbers and my age, I would be a perfect candidate for IVF.

I was stunned at the fact that I had to go to the length of resorting to drastic measures to conceive a baby. On a second thought, I started getting excited about it. I visualized myself getting pregnant and having a baby, and it felt so good. Finally, all the hospital visits, blood tests, countless invasive ultrasounds, medications, trigger injections, timed intercourse, mood swings, sadness, and so on would come to an end with this one giant step. If IVF was the magic pill that would release me from the bondage of struggling with fertility, I was more than happy to get it done. I was so enthusiastic about it.

Prior to my journey, I had only heard a thing or two about ARTs in general, and all along I believed using ARTs as a means to achieve a pregnancy was the one-shot silver-bullet fertility challenge solution and a gateway to having multiples in one go. I had no idea that in actuality, it is a nail-biting situation—until I started getting deeper into the process and learning more about all the dynamics involved. The more informed I became, the more terrified I grew.

Doing IVF is definitely not a guarantee that you will get pregnant, and even if you do get pregnant, it is not guaranteed that you will have a baby. That's the sad truth I wasn't well informed about until ARTs became my reality. I could not comprehend the fact that with all that my body had to go through, there was even the slightest possibility that I might have a big, fat negative pregnancy test in the end. With this new and not-so-pleasing information, we crossed everything we had and decided to proceed with the journey, hoping for the best. The good thing is that it didn't feel obligatory. It felt like it was the right thing to do in our quest for a baby.

In light of the above, we set out on a search for a fertility clinic abroad that would meet our needs. This was actually a very challenging part of the process. We sent out inquiries to as many fertility centers as we possibly could in an effort to find the best. Comparing the responses we received from these centers, we realized that they all offered almost the same kind of services, making it very tough to arrive at a decision as to which center to choose. After detailed consultation sessions, we finally picked out a center to work with. But wait … There is more! Picking out a center doesn't mean that center will accept you as a patient.

First, you must meet their acceptance criteria to be guaranteed treatment. During preliminary tests and screening consultations with the fertility doctor, we discussed my medical history and my husband's as well. The doctor requested results of my hormonal tests, ovarian assessments, and semen analysis from my husband. Although I had them handy, she preferred to rerun these tests at their clinic, which was fine with us. Oh, did I just say fine with us? Ignore that It was fine with me but not with Tim, as he dislikes giving semen samples. Too bad. There wasn't really any choice here. He had to do it. Poor thing! The thought of it made him sick.

In case you didn't know, almost everything with ARTs in general is time-sensitive. Certain tests can only be done during a particular window in a woman's cycle or else you get inaccurate and misleading results. That said, we had to wait for day two of my cycle in order to get my tests done. (You probably remember this trend from phase 1.) The sixteen-day wait literally felt like sixteen weeks. At least I had firsthand background knowledge on this from my past medicated but non-IVF cycles. Day two is the magical day where blood is drawn to run all necessary tests before engaging in any procedure. They have to make sure your numbers are at their right levels for the procedure, and samples taken on day two tend to give doctors exactly what they are looking for.

Day two finally arrived, and our tests were done. At approximately a quarter past four on a Tuesday afternoon, we got a call from one of the nurses at the clinic with news that our test results were in and we could come in later that evening to meet with the doctor to discuss the results. She had a 6:30 p.m. slot available, which worked perfectly well for a working couple like us, so we jumped on it. At the appointment, the fertility doctor discussed our results and told us they were happy with our numbers and would be pleased to work with us. She equally discussed a recommended personalized treatment program reached from our results and unique circumstances.

Following all preliminary tests and clearances, we were officially ready to embark on our unique IVF journey. IVF is a very exciting but equally daunting and emotional journey. In my case, the excitement emanated from the end results of the process. I would finally get the long-awaited positive pregnancy test and a baby in my arms nine months down the road. This got me really excited. On the other hand, there were a lot of mixed emotions running through me as I underwent this process. (You will learn more about it as things unfold in subsequent paragraphs.)

In a woman's natural monthly cycle, her ovaries normally produce one egg, but with a medicated or stimulated cycle, the medications encourage the follicles in her ovaries to produce multiple eggs. The medications they use contain hormones, with the most common ones being the follicle-stimulating hormone (FSH) and the luteinizing hormone (LH). These are hormones that are produced naturally in the body at the right levels when everything is working the way it should. When there is a shift of any kind and these hormones are imbalanced, medications and injections are needed to boost the natural levels to encourage more eggs to develop.

When I started my stimulation phase of this process, I had no idea what I had signed up for. It was approximately two weeks of one to two injections per day coupled with a lot of pills to take in order to stimulate my ovaries. There were constant blood tests and multiple transvaginal ultrasounds in order to monitor the ovaries and the development of the follicles to make any adjustments to medications and dosages if need be.

The good thing is that my hotel was only a two-minute walk to the clinic, which wasn't only convenient but equally saved me the trouble of having to inject myself every single day as other patients do during this process. It can be a very daunting task. I took advantage of this and had the nurses do the job for me. Patients who lived far away or those who had to go to work didn't have this kind of luxury. They had to either bite the bullet and give themselves the injections daily or rope their partners or friends into doing it for them.

Toward the end of the stimulation phase, things got intense. I was monitored more frequently. This phase (like many others) is a very important phase in the IVF process because the medical team has to time the trigger injection (it gets the eggs ready for ovulation) perfectly. Remember that time-sensitive thing we talked about in previous paragraphs? Timing is very critical during this process, and they take it very seriously. Considering all the hard work that the medical team has put in to get me to this point coupled with everything my body, mind, and soul has been through, it would be horrific if they missed this critical step.

Once my follicles were spotted to have advanced to the right size, the trigger shot was administered, and I was given strict instructions on what to do and when to be back at the clinic for the egg pickup/collection/retrieval procedure. It is carefully timed so that the retrieval is done right before you are due to ovulate. Egg pickup/collection/retrieval is a delicate twenty- to thirty-minute procedure under twilight anesthesia (a medication-induced sleep during which you breathe on your own) wherein a needle is carefully guided through the vagina into each ovary to collect the fluid within the follicles that contain the eggs.

As soon as we arrived at the clinic (the morning of the egg retrieval), my husband gave a fresh semen sample to be introduced into the eggs that would be collected from my ovaries. Prior to this procedure, the doctor had given us a fair idea of how many eggs to expect to be gleaned based on the ultrasounds she performed. We had about a dozen eggs developing pleasingly, which was great. Great not because we wanted a dozen babies, but great because it gave us hope of success. With a dozen eggs, there is a decent chance that at least a handful will fertilize and become embryos. This definitely made it easier to go through some extremely draining days filled with tons of emotions.

After the procedure was over, I felt a little bit groggy and fatigued from the anesthesia but nothing ghastly. It took approximately fifty minutes for me to recover and receive the doctor's clearance to go home. I recovered nicely and was able to walk on my own without any pain. Before we left the clinic, we were told that twelve eggs were retrieved and had been sent to the lab to be cultured. We were also given detailed post-op instructions on what to do each and every step of the way.

I still remember how ecstatic I was to have made it to this stage and how I couldn't stop thinking about the babies we would have from this process. I was so delighted that I cried. I envisioned us with our baby, and life never felt so perfect. I was looking forward to having our little embryos being put back into me and growing bigger and bigger by the day. All those frustrations with timed medications and a great loss of privacy were gradually turning into joy. The focus was gradually shifting to a bigger, better, and more positive picture.

The next day, we got a call with details on the final number of eggs that were deemed mature. Within the next few days, we were constantly being updated on the progress of our eggs, sperm, and embryo development. Overall, they were doing fantastic, and it was determined from this that we could either benefit from a day three or day five embryo transfer. We opted for a day five transfer because we found comfort in knowing that our embryos would have made it to the blastocysts stage and because we believed that implanting embryos at that stage into the uterus often boosts chances of a successful pregnancy. We were also briefed on what we needed to do to prepare for the procedure.

Unlike the egg retrieval (ER), I found the embryo transfer (ET) to be very complex and nerve-wracking. Although it is a simple, five-minute procedure that can be likened to a Pap smear, it wasn't as straightforward as the ER procedure in my humble opinion. With the ER procedure, all I had to do was to refrain from eating or drinking the night before and come in wearing comfortable clothing with no perfume, makeup, or contact lenses. The thirty-minute procedure was more about the medical team doing their job and less about what I had to do to make their job more efficient, effective, and successful.

On the other hand of the equation lies the ET with taxing do's and don'ts. First, I was instructed to arrive at my appointment with a full bladder. Initially, it sounded quite easy, but the more I thought about it, the more intricate it appeared. How full is considered full? I struggled with this requirement tremendously. I feared that my transfer might not be successful because I didn't have the right amount of liquid in my bladder. I knew that it would be monitored to make sure the amount was right, but I was still troubled about this.

To make matters worse, I did myself a great disservice by engaging in a lengthy chitchat session with a lady who was going through IVF for the fourth time, with three failed previous cycles. As you may have gathered from previous chapters in this book, it is easier to chat freely about fertility struggles and IVF with those who are going through it because you feel very secure with them. You let your guard down and express yourself the best you can without any fear of being judged, labeled, or shamed.

As much as I enjoyed my chats with this lady, this particular conversation left me in shambles. Simply mentioning the fact that my egg retrieval had been scheduled for the next day sprang in her a scary amount of advice to give to me about taking the full bladder requirement very seriously. Among a host of things she said, I couldn't stop thinking about her saying that people have had their cycles cancelled because they didn't fulfill this minor but very essential requirement and that some transfers have failed for the same reason. This lady scared me to death and got me scrambling for my mobile device in order to conduct some quick research and find ways to circumvent ruining my ET.

Turning to the internet was such an awful idea, as I ended up aggravating my already messed-up psyche by reading negative things I never should have read. If I had to advise you, I would give you a stern warning to avoid the internet as much as you can when going through IVF. In as much as it is good to educate yourself, there is a lot of unverified information on the internet that will confuse you, stress you out, and distract you from your objective. Here I was on the eve of my ET as confused as a homeless man on house arrest. This is definitely not an ideal situation. I was a complete nervous wreck. My husband (bless him) tried all he could to calm me down, which helped enormously in getting me through the night.

Mindful of the fact that a full bladder is a crucial factor of the ET process, as it facilitates the visualization of the uterus by abdominal ultrasound and causes reflex nervous suppression of the uterine contractility, I ended up drinking more water than I was supposed to. (I wouldn't be surprised if you predicted this catastrophe already.) This made me so uncomfortable to the point where I had to empty my bladder right before I was called up to be prepped for the procedure. Who does that? Anyway, this set me back a whole hour, as I had to wait for my bladder to fill up again.

While waiting, I drank on some more water to facilitate the bladder fill-up process. As I waited, I listened for every drop into my bladder. Gradually, I began feeling some pressure, which was a good indicator that I was getting there. I updated the nurse, and she took me in, monitored my progress, and prepped me for the procedure once she spotted on the ultrasound that my bladder had filled up to the right level. She could see everything on the monitor. I could even see it for myself too. My bladder was full!

As I laid down and began chatting to the nurse, the doctor walked in with the rest of her team with big, bright smiles on their faces, ready to perform my final procedure. So much preparation had led up to this moment. The medical team had worked tirelessly, and I had been through weeks of medications and injections, countless ultrasounds, the ER procedure, and the waiting period for the embryos to be cultured in the lab. It was so surreal to finally be in the moment when our precious embryos would be introduced into my uterus. For me, this was the most exciting and most emotional moment of my entire IVF cycle.

As the doctor and her team fiddled with all kinds of medical equipment and medical parlance here and there, I hoped and anticipated for the best. The procedure doesn't require any anesthetic or sedation, so I was awake the entire time and lived the moment firsthand. It was a relatively easy and simple process compared to some of the procedures I've been through prior in my quest for a baby. Guided by an ultrasound, which I watched the entire time, the doctor used a fine transfer catheter to meticulously move our embryos through my vagina and cervix into my uterus. It was a very short, straightforward, and pain-free procedure.

After the procedure, I continued to lie on my back for another forty-five minutes in the recovery room before being released. I took the rest of the day off and did nothing. I took it easy on myself and truly relaxed for once since we had engaged on this journey.

Why was I so nervous the previous day and even in the moments leading up to this procedure? Why did I put myself through the trauma? It wasn't worth it. In hindsight, I had no business stressing myself out the way I did. But again, with IVF, it's hard to think straight. You just have to dig your heels in and roll with the punches.

While some doctors do recommend bed rest for twenty-four hours after the procedure, some do not, and there is actually no evidence that proves it is necessary to be on rest post-ET. Other sources suggest that you can resume your normal daily activities, as moving around may enhance blood flow to the uterus. The truth is that it probably doesn't matter whether you choose to go on bed rest. What matters is that you heed to your doctor's advice, listen to your body, and do what feels right. If you feel too tired, it might be an indication that you need to give yourself some time to relax. If you feel anxious with the urge to move, it might not be a dreadful idea to take a gentle walk around to help relieve some of the stress. Whatever the case maybe, keep your doctor informed, and do right by your body.

Two days after the procedure, I flew back home and resumed my normal activities while waiting for the two-week wait to elapse in order for me to take my pregnancy test. I must confess that patience was extremely difficult during this period. My mind has never been so curios. It kept asking whether I was pregnant, and I couldn't wait to find out. To be quite candid, I totally believed I was pregnant, but I wanted the confirmation in order to ease my nerves.

Following the procedure, I had been counseled not to test during the two-week wait because the hormone used to trigger ovulation right before ER is the same hormone used to measure pregnancy in home pregnancy tests. This hormone can linger in your bloodstream for a good while before wearing off, which means you risk getting misleading results should you test too early. In some cases, you could be pregnant but with very low HCG to register on the test. In such situations, you will get a false negative if you test too early. Getting a false negative leaves you stressed out, and getting a false positive just to find out down the road that you aren't really pregnant could be very emotionally daunting. It is best to wait it out and go in for your beta test as scheduled if you want accurate results.

While waiting, I took my post-procedure medications religiously and ate a healthy diet. My diet consisted of a lot of protein, fiber, and vegetables. I stayed away from potential risky foods, avoided vigorous exercises, drank lots of water, and got plenty of sleep. I tried my best to take it easy on myself and to keep a positive mindset. Eating a healthy diet came naturally to me because that's part of my lifestyle, but staying positive after coming to the realization that IVF is not guaranteed was a challenging factor. I battled with negative thoughts and a whole lot of anxiety during this period. After all that had been vested in the process, it was hard to not hope for the best but fear for the worst.

Another challenging factor that we faced during the wait had to do with administering my injections. I had gotten so used to walking to the clinic and having the nurses do that job for me while abroad. It was so much easier that way. I hate needles and never want to look at them. But here I had no choice. Before flying back home, we took a crash course on administering injections. Everything looked so easy on the surface until it was time to get the job done. My husband started administering the injections for me, but it became too emotional.

Watching him do it was ripping me apart, but I wasn't mentally ready or capable of injecting myself, so again, I had to roll with the punches. One morning, I braved myself in the bathroom and took the injection all by myself. I couldn't believe I actually just injected myself. From then onward, I got increasingly comfortable at doing it and eventually became an expert. My fear of needles was gradually suppressed, and I survived the remainder of the process. It truly always seems impossible until it is done. Who knew that I could ever touch needles and syringes, let alone inject myself?

During this excruciating two-week wait, I experienced—or maybe thought I experienced—all kinds of pregnancy symptoms. With IVF, you are in a different special world carefully crafted for you, so you tend to feel things that do not even exist. I felt a baby moving in my stomach during the two-week wait. Sometimes I felt one, and sometimes I felt two. I was so convinced I had two babies in me. It's weird because with my first natural pregnancy, I didn't even know I was pregnant until I missed a period, and even when I found out I was pregnant, I didn't feel any quickening until I was about sixteen weeks along.

Clearly, those movements I felt during the two-week wait were all in my head. On the flip side, there were some actual symptoms during the wait. I felt extremely bloated and fatigued and had sore breasts. I also experienced a lot of mood swings. One minute I would be so happy, the next I was grumpy and ugly crying for no reason, the next I was happy again, and before you know it, I was snapping at everyone around me. All of these happened abruptly and uncontrollably and solidified and anchored my thinking into believing I was pregnant.

Approximately two weeks after my transfer, I went in for my blood test to determine whether I was pregnant but really hoping that I was pregnant. Low and behold, I got a call later that afternoon with news that there wasn't really any HCG in my bloodstream, meaning I wasn't pregnant. I was completely devastated and heartbroken. My IVF cycle had failed. How disappointing! It literally felt like bereavement. I had lost the child I envisioned.

I thought about how I watched the embryos being transferred into my uterus during my ET procedure. I remembered the movements I felt during the two-week wait. I was in a trance for a while. I was convinced the entire time that I would end up with two or at least one baby from this process. It never really crossed my mind that we would come out with none. I could feel renewed grief and distress caressing my being. I could feel it deep in my soul. In that moment, my thoughts went wild, and I found myself reminiscing some important uplifting moments and dark sorrowful events.

I pictured each and every step of the process from the time I was told I would be a good candidate for IVF to the time I got on the plane to fly abroad for treatment.

I pictured how excited I was when I received the first stimulation injection to the time my follicles were ready to be triggered.

I pictured the egg retrieval and the embryo transfer procedures.

I pictured the loss of privacy to countless invasive ultrasound procedures.

I pictured the crash course on administering injections.

I pictured the drive to the airport and the flight back home.

I pictured my husband injecting me and how meticulous he did it.

I pictured me injecting myself.

I pictured my medications and the massive medical supply box.

I pictured my scar from my emergency C-section.

I pictured my growing belly from my natural spontaneous pregnancy.

I pictured myself in the ambulance on August 4, 2014.

I pictured myself holding my beautiful stillborn baby boy.

I pictured myself fighting for my life after the C-section with little to no blood left in me.

I pictured myself in the hospital hallway in that hospital gown learning how to walk again.

I pictured myself picking out what my angel baby would wear to be laid to rest.

I pictured myself watching him being lowered deep into the ground.

I pictured everything.

How do I move forward given my circumstances? Regroup and try again or throw in the towel and accept that I wasn't cut out to birth a child? Was it time to draw the hard line? Will I be giving up if I draw the hard line? These are questions that I'm still trying to figure out answers to. And to be quite transparent, I haven't found any good answers … just yet. I know for a fact that I will make a good mother to my children; however, I do not know what my route to motherhood is destined to be.

If I had the answer to this fundamental question, it would be a lot easier to think through the issues and embark on a journey with a guaranteed outcome. For the lack of this vital knowledge, I will continue to soar and fight for my fertility with everything I've got in order to give myself the deserving satisfaction that I did everything I could to make it happen; I tried my best—my very best. To me, failure has never been an option and will never be an option.

To sum it all up, IVF was a huge eye-opener for me. No matter the amount of research I did, it remained a learn-as-you-go process. There was always something new. I learned to take one step at a time, putting one foot in front of the other. After suffering my loss, I hit rock bottom as detailed in phase 1 of this book. That loss zapped a lot of energy out of me—so much such that I hardly believed I had any strength left until IVF became my reality.

Going through the process and ending up with a big fat negative pregnancy test and still being able to continue to pursue life is proof to me that I am resilient, strong, and determined. With every disappointment, I have learned to pause, take a deep breath, and concentrate on the next step. I no longer pride myself in setting time lines and goals on baby making that I will almost undoubtedly fail to achieve. This can break me, and I cannot afford to break. I have to do everything possible to protect my sanity, accept my reality, and enjoy life.

Fertility treatment is a significant emotional journey. Being new to the process and having no one to truly talk to was emotionally exhausting and devastating. It's just not something people talk about with a group of friends over brunch. The majority suffer in silence not because they want to but because fertility struggles carry a huge stigma. You truly don't realize how stigmatized this topic is until it becomes your reality. It takes a lot to stay focused and continue with your daily activities while feeling completely wrecked on the inside. Thankfully, we managed to sail through it somehow without losing our minds.

CHAPTER 2

Public Figures on Fertility Struggles

As earlier mentioned, high-profile people also suffer their own emotional difficulties, but just a few of them are bold enough to speak up about it, and that too is OK because it takes a lot to be able to talk about these things. Below you will find a combination of diverse but great analogies of fertility struggles faced by some public figures who have been brave enough to come forward and share their unique fertility battles with the world.

A special thank you to these strong, fearless, and inspiring women for putting their names and faces to this stigmatized topic. Given the fact that they have a huge platform to reach out and inspire, I wish for them to continue to speak up about this taboo so that, together, we can demystify the stigma and free up those who are still struggling in hiding.

Gabrielle Union

This powerhouse of a woman has been very open about her fertility journey. She has gone on air several times on different platforms and spoken about her struggle to become a mom and how she suffered multiple miscarriages in the process. She has opened up about being in rooms at fertility doctors' offices with other women suffering the same fate, but at the same time, there is such a shroud of secrecy and shame among these women.

She's even made mention of the fact that there are back entrances and people who will come get you from your car with an umbrella, so people don't see you going to the office of a fertility doctor. She continues to articulate that she would rather be the guinea pig and speak about the process to demystify the stigma and save as many people as she can.

Chrissy Teigen

It is no secret that Chrissy does not bite her tongue when it comes to her battle with fertility. She said that if they were not having trouble conceiving, they would have had their kids many years ago. She acknowledges that it was a process for them and that they saw fertility doctors. She has said that once you begin to open up about your struggles to other people, that's when you start learning that a lot of other people in your life are visiting fertility doctors and have this shame about it.

Built on their struggles, she says, "So anytime somebody asks me if I'm going to have kids, I'm like, one day, you're going to ask that to the wrong girl who is really struggling, and it's going to be really hurtful to them. And I hate that. So, I hate it. Stop asking me!"

Wendy Williams

The talk show host who is a mother of one has also braved it and spoken about her journey with fertility. She doesn't shy away from talking about the many miscarriages she suffered, including two at five months. At this point, they had the clothes already picked out, and the nursery was already painted just to end up losing the pregnancy and being faced with questions such as: Do you want a funeral, or do you want a cremation? Wendy shared that they went through this struggle more than twice.

She is grateful for her son and views him as a hard-won child. She says, "I would've loved to have had more children, but I don't want to test my blessing. Being a mother is for me. It's not for everybody. It's for me."

Kim Kardashian

Kim, the influential *Keeping Up with the Kardashian* star has been very open about her fertility journey on the show and on other platforms as much as she can. However, she articulates that she didn't know that she was going to be so open with her fertility challenges. But meeting people at her fertility doctor's office who were going through the same things she was going through got her thinking, why not share her story with the world?

She said, "It's been really emotional. One doctor told me I would need my uterus removed after I had another baby—I could only have one more. One was like, 'You should get a surrogate.' The other one was like, 'Oh, no, you'll be fine.' Then I called my doctor, and he's like, 'You know what? I believe—we'll get through it.'"

She has also shared that there were definitely times when she walked out of the doctor's office hysterically crying, and other times when she walked out feeling that everything was looking good and hoping that she would get a positive pregnancy test during that cycle.

Celine Dion

Renowned for her powerful, technically skilled vocals, the best-selling Canadian recording artist with record sales of more than two hundred million worldwide let slip that she too struggled with fertility issues. Precisely, she did IVF six times, one after the other before falling pregnant with her twins. Celine has been very vocal about the fact that so long as her health permitted her to keep going or unless her doctor told her that she couldn't physically handle IVF anymore, she would have kept going until she achieved a pregnancy. She acknowledged the fact that some people stop because it is a very expensive procedure; however, she kept going while trying to relax and stay positive.

When this superstar talks about her struggle with fertility, she often explains how it affected not only her personal life but her work as well. Torn between her career and building a family, or a life and a contract as she prefers to word it, she made the choice to hit the pause button on her contract. She details that she was not going to stop just because she had a contract for singing and that she would have hated every song she sang for the rest of her life if she had chosen to put her baby quest journey on hold. As a result, she asked for the Caesars Palace shows to be postponed because it just wasn't a good enough reason for her not to try for a baby.

Angela Bassett

Angela Evelyn Bassett, the incredibly talented movie star, director, producer, activist, and mother of two has had her own share of the fertility struggle pie. Opening up about her battles with fertility, she shared that after trying and trying, she unfortunately couldn't birth her own babies. According to her, "It was my reality. I heard about the surrogate option and it worked out beautifully."

Beyoncé

One of the world's best-selling recording artists with more than 118 million records sold worldwide coupled with at least twenty-eight Grammy Awards and a host of other impressive accolades, Beyonce Giselle Knowles Carter was faced with fertility challenges when it came to time to start and grow her family and has been very open about those struggles.

When she finally succeeded in getting pregnant for the first time, she was delighted. She said the sound of her baby's heartbeat was the most beautiful music she's ever heard in her life. She went ahead and picked out names and envisioned what her child would look like and was feeling very maternal. One day she went in for her routine examination, and there was no heartbeat. Her baby was gone, and she was devastated and qualifies this as the saddest thing she has ever been through. As a coping mechanism, she went into the studio and wrote the saddest song she's ever written in her entire life.

Giuliana Rancic

Giuliana, the Italian American entertainment reporter, television personality, and coanchor of *E News* was fearless to have shared her fertility battle on air in the reality television show *Giuliana and Bill*. She disclosed that after their third round of IVF, they successfully had embryos to transfer back into her; however, that process could not be completed because it was discovered that she had breast cancer. With part of the treatment being five years of tamoxifen, which can cause birth defects, their next reasonable available option was to consider using a surrogate, which worked out perfectly, and they welcomed a baby boy named Duke some nine months later.

Elizabeth Banks

Being a movie star and playing Effie Trinket in the *Hunger Games* film series doesn't mean you will escape fertility challenges. Elizabeth Banks has a fertility journey story too and has been generous enough to be open about it. She had issues with her womb that were preventing embryos from implanting.

She revealed that she had to use a surrogate in order to become a mom when she said, "It's a big leap, inviting this person into your life to do this amazing, important thing for you. And it's hard losing that kind of control. But our surrogate is so extraordinary, and she's still in our lives. She's like an auntie."

Nicole Kidman

The Australian actress, producer, and singer who has bagged several awards, including, but not limited to, at least five Golden Globe Awards, two Primetime Emmy Awards, and an Academy Award, has also suffered fertility issues. Speaking up about these challenges, the top Hollywood import feels like anyone who has been in the place of wanting a child and knows the disappointment, the pain, and the loss that you go through trying and struggling with fertility.

She thinks "fertility is such a big thing, and it's not something I've ever run away from talking about. We were in a place of desperately wanting another child. I couldn't get pregnant. Our surrogate was the most wonderful woman to do this for us. I get emotional talking about it because I'm so grateful to her."

Sarah Jessica Parker

Known for her role as Carrie Bradshaw on the HBO television series *Sex and the City*, this brilliant American actress and producer encountered fertility challenges while trying to have children. She revealed that she tried so hard to get pregnant, but it just wasn't going to happen the conventional, predictable way. She had her children via surrogate, and while she cherished all the milestones, the good and the bad, she acknowledges that meeting her children rather than giving birth to them felt like a suspended animation. You miss out on the gestational experience, and it is as if everything else disappears for a moment, and the world goes silent. Although having babies through the eccentric way is different, Sarah Jessica Parker thinks it is equally extraordinary and amazing.

Mariah Carey

Noted for her remarkable vocal range, the American pop star has also had to fight for her fertility and has been brave enough to talk about it openly. She declared that their struggle shook them and took them into a place that was really dark and difficult, adding that, "When that happened … I wasn't able to even talk to anybody about it. That was not easy."

Michelle Obama

Lying comfortably on a cream-white microfiber sofa couch in my living room on the evening of Saturday, November 9, 2018, I picked up my rose-gold iPhone 6S Plus device to catch up on the news via news flash, something I do almost on a daily basis because my days are often so filled, leaving me with very little to no time to watch television or even to listen to the news. Swiping my thumb from bottom to top over and over again, I saw a captivating headline that read: "Dispelling taboos, Michelle Obama talks IVF and miscarriage." Being a person who was currently struggling with fertility, had been through IVF, and was in the process of telling my story, I couldn't let this pass by.

I quickly clicked on the link to educate myself with Michelle's ever-so-wise, educative, and encouraging words. Astonishingly, it wasn't some general talk. The first lady was actually getting real, going so deep and personal about her own struggles with fertility, opening up about her miscarriage and how she relied on IVF to conceive her two beautiful daughters. I did not see this coming. "Wow! Michelle Obama?" I exclaimed. I was so excited and even more propelled to read about it all—another high-profile individual putting her name and face to the fertility struggle picture collage.

This time around, it was not a Hollywood star; it was Michelle Obama, the former first lady of the United States of America, the greatest country in the world. "Wow! This is going to be remarkable," I said to myself. It is important to indicate that at this moment, I was in the second proofreading phase of this book, and I was happy with the content and convinced I wouldn't be adding any more text to it. Guess what? I was completely wrong. Michelle's revelation instantly rubbed off the giant full stop I had placed on this chapter in particular and on the book in general. I knew I had to include her revelation.

I dropped everything, climbed off of my couch, scrambled for my jet-black eighteen-inch Hewlett-Packard Pavilion, and sat at the table. As soon as the computer powered on, I looked up the interview with Robin Roberts on the CNN website that had aired on *Good Morning America* (*GMA*). I wanted to watch it and see for myself in order to avoid any diluted information from online sources.

The former first lady told Robin Roberts on the Friday, November 8, 2018, interview on *Good Morning America* that: "I felt lost and alone and I felt like I failed." She also said, "I didn't know how common miscarriages were because we don't talk about them. We sit in our own pain thinking that somehow we are broken." She added that she felt "lost and alone" after having a miscarriage twenty years ago and had to do IVF to conceive her daughters.

After all is said and done, Michelle thinks the worst thing we do to each other as women is "not share the truth about our bodies and how they work and how they don't work." I couldn't agree more! Like the adage goes, information is power. Do you have the courage to use your experience to educate that young girl or that woman next to you?

I can't really articulate exactly how I felt after watching this interview, but I can tell you there was an uplifting thing that happened to me. And this is exactly how I always feel whenever a public figure speaks up about her fertility struggles and how it affected or still affects her life. The former first lady (just like the other incredible ladies mentioned above) really did open herself up to the world in bold ways. She touched on other very important subject matters in her memoire, but this one piece of her journey about struggling with fertility resonates with me.

Fertility struggles is a subject that's very close to my heart, yet one that often remains in the shadows because it carries a stigma. Mrs. Obama, like many other women out there (including myself), have suffered in silence. This reminds me that I'm not alone and that it is not happening because of me; it is happening to me. As a matter of fact, she underwent these procedures twenty years ago and is only able to speak up about it now. This portrays the emotional impact it had or has on her and how heavy the consequences of struggling with fertility are on those dealing with it or on those who've had to deal with it at some point in their lives.

Coincidentally, I had read a post that same Friday morning, November 8, 2018, on social media about Gabrielle Union and her basketball superstar husband, Dwayne Wade, welcoming a baby girl via surrogate. In that joyful post, there were beautiful skin-to-skin pictures of mother and father bonding with their beautiful newborn baby girl. Knowing Gabby's struggle with fertility, I was ecstatic for her and couldn't wait to read the entire post. Despondently, one of the first comments I read was: "Why are they faking pictures when the baby was born via surrogate?" I froze for a long minute, completely bewildered by what I had just read. I couldn't comprehend such insensitivity.

I was so upset and filled with so much fury and profanity toward this individual who happened to be a complete stranger. I literally had to practice a great deal of self-control in order not to touch my keyboard and lash out at this individual with horrendous words. After giving it a second thought, it occurred to me that this individual might actually not have an understanding of what surrogacy means because if he did, he wouldn't say such horrifying things to someone trying to bond with their baby. This really just reiterated the fact that we need to create more awareness about fertility struggles.

There are also people who are fully aware and well informed on surrogacy and what it entails, but still, they choose to not fully accept babies born via such means as they do with a baby conceived and born through the predictable way. To these people, I can only hope that one day they will understand the dynamics and challenges of fertility and be more open and accepting of parents and their babies born via assisted reproductive technologies. While hoping, we must continue to enlighten, educate, and inspire those around us the best we can.

Michelle's revelation gives me hope that one day, this topic will no longer be in the shadows, and people like the insensitive one mentioned above will be more educated about fertility and its challenges, regardless of whether they are affected by it. I also hope that with such a revelation coming from a high-profile lady with a high-profile name and face, the conversations that surround this topic will shift gears to a positive direction where people who've been fortunate enough to be spared this kind of struggle will perhaps learn to be more understanding, more empathetic, and more careful with their word choices when carrying on conversations with the affected—one that removes stigmas and uplifts those affected. I wish for this powerful revelation to not only serve as an informant to the world about her struggles but truly serve as an eye-opener and a massive tool to help those fighting for their fertility.

Researching further, I stumbled upon some very educational remarks by the incredible Dr. Zev Williams, director of the Columbia University Fertility Center and coauthor of the 2015 study: "Looking into Public Perceptions of Miscarriage."

In this study, he articulated that, "There is a real sense of self-blame and guilt and a reluctance to discuss it with other people." In discussing miscarriage, he says miscarriage or pregnancy loss occurs in at least twenty percent of all pregnancies, and 55 percent of those who responded to his survey thought miscarriage was a rare thing, occurring in only 5 percent or less of pregnancies. Some believed that they occur in less than 0.1 percent. What a remarkable difference between the perceived and actual figures. He further articulated that, "Of those who had a miscarriage, 37% reported feeling that they had lost a child, 47% felt guilty, 41% reported feeling that they had done something wrong, 41% felt alone, and 28% felt ashamed."

Do you realize that no positive feeling was reported by the women who undertook the survey? I don't think it happened by coincidence. There is nothing positive about a miscarriage or pregnancy loss or fertility struggles. If anything, it leaves the affected feeling a sense of loss, self-blame, guilt, shame, and loneliness. Dr. Zev also brought forward the fact that not only are miscarriages common across the globe, but they are also in most cases not the mother's fault, and the fact that this kind of information is not widely known only makes matters worse. Statistics even report that since Louise Brown, the first IVF baby born in 1978, more than eight million children have been born via IVF worldwide. People struggle to have babies. The narrative around this topic has to change.

With the above, you'd think the stigma should be long gone by now, but no. It is still strongly present and affecting millions of people across the globe. It is sad that even with available conspicuous statistics, the fertility topic is still one with a stigma. Many people battling with their fertility keep their feelings and struggles under wraps, trying to cope alone and withering in excruciating pain. A significant number of fertility specialists confirm that couples dealing with fertility struggles more often than not tend to conceal their struggles.

In one survey of couples who were having difficulties to conceive, 61 percent said they had not discussed their struggles with family and friends, and nearly half of them said they had not even discussed the issue with their own mothers. Sad, isn't it? People shouldn't feel bad to talk about important things like this. They shouldn't shy away from it. They shouldn't be shrouded in misery and shame for something they didn't do to themselves and something they have absolutely no control over whatsoever.

Fertility struggle is a massively misunderstood disease, and sadly, it affects approximately one in every eight couples, and these couples need help in dealing with the consequences of this disease just like any other disease out there. It's a shame that although the World Health Organization (WHO) has recognized struggles with fertility as a physical illness that requires treatment, society still doesn't. We need to raise more awareness about the pain these challenges bring because it is a very serious disease, and society needs to understand its scale and ramifications.

While I am incredibly impressed and proud of the above-mentioned brave women who mustered up the courage to share their stories with the world, I would love to see a multidimensional representation of women on mainstream media sharing their stories on this topic. We need a representation with diverse people, diverse context, and diverse stories, not just high-profile people.

It's about finding the value, validity, and courage in each and every person's story, irrespective of her social or financial status in society. If we can do this, I believe that would be a valuable and giant step toward challenging and shattering the stigma that continues to surround pregnancy loss and infertility. We can do better, and we should do better.

CHAPTER 3

Who Does This Disease Affect?

The struggle with fertility does not discriminate. It can affect anyone who falls within childbearing age. It affects people all over the world across all walks of life. It affects both men and women. In the United States alone, the Centers for Disease Control and Prevention reports that about 12 percent of women (7.4 million) and 9 percent of men within reproductive ages have been affected by this disease at some point in their lives.

According to the US Department of Health and Human Services, a whopping 6.1 million women out of the 7.4 million suffer from polycystic ovarian syndrome (PCOS), making it the most common cause of female fertility struggles. Within the remaining 1.3 million people, some suffer from various medically diagnosed conditions, while others suffer from an unidentifiable cause.

Predicated on reports gathered from the American Society for Reproductive Medicine and data from National Health Statistic Reports, 12 to 15 percent of couples are unable to conceive after one year of having unprotected sex. Even after two years, 10 percent of these couples are still not successful in having a baby. Although fertility declines with age and women are about half as fertile in their thirties as they were in their twenties, you will be amazed by the following statistics.

Generally, in healthy couples who are younger than thirty, only 40 to 60 percent are able to conceive after three months of trying. It takes longer for about 40 percent of these younger and healthy couples even with assisted reproduction technologies. The struggle with fertility is real and must not be overlooked.

In my fertility journey, I met people from all walks of life battling similar struggles. I met lawyers, doctors, business owners, nurses, accountants, engineers, pharmacists, teachers, bankers, psychologists, administrators, motivational speakers, top executives, and much more. I met girls as young as eighteen and ladies as old as fifty-three. It was such an eye-opener and an invaluable learning experience for me. I would never have believed the above statistics if I hadn't gone through this journey. Who would have thought that an eighteen-year-old would be struggling with fertility?

The majority of young adults believe that struggling with fertility is something that surfaces with age. No! That's a huge misconception. It is not always about age. As mentioned earlier, the struggle with fertility does not discriminate. You don't have to be a geriatric to be on fertility struggle bus. So long as you fall within childbearing age, you can be susceptible to fertility struggles. Sadly, in our society, you only begin to learn about these truths once you've already been diagnosed with the disease, and at that point, it is too late and overwhelming.

Most adolescents must have heard of the word *infertility* but never associate it with themselves. They think it's something only for those aged thirty-five and older to be concerned about. Think of what would happen if more awareness were created. We need to educate people about fertility as much as we can. When equipped with the right information, our decision-making process about important things gets so much easier.

If I knew what I know today when I was an adolescent, I would have done things differently for myself. Now I know better, but there isn't much I can do to help myself. The good news is that although I cannot help myself, I can use what I have experienced and learned to educate, encourage, and help others. The struggle with fertility poses as a monster with horrendous consequences, and I do not wish that on anyone because I know the pain and how emotionally devastating it can be to patients and their partners.

CHAPTER 4

Fertility Struggle Consequences

The psychological challenges faced by women receiving fertility advice or treatment are far more common but usually private. While the consequences of this disease are overwhelmingly physiological, the resulting headache, often exacerbated by the physical and emotional rigors of treatment, may exact a huge psychological toll on patients. For example, during one study of two hundred couples who were seen consecutively at a fertility clinic, it was discovered that half of the women and 15 percent of the men when asked about struggling with fertility said it was the most upsetting experience of their lives.

In another study of approximately five hundred American women who filled out a standard psychological questionnaire before undergoing a stress reduction, it was concluded that women struggling with fertility felt as anxious or as depressed as those battling cancer and hypertension or those recovering from a heart attack.

Significantly less research has been carried out to rate men's reactions to fertility struggles, but in the few that have been done, they generally tend to report experiencing less distress when compared to women. However, their reactions depend on whether they or their partners are diagnosed with the disease. In most cases, when the female partner is the one diagnosed with the disease, men do not report being as anxious and as distressed as the women, most especially because they have to be strong for their partners. On the flip side, when men get the news that they've been diagnosed, they experience the same levels of anxiety, depression, stigma, and low self-esteem as women struggling with infertility.

In my fertility journey, I met and interacted with countless couples struggling with their fertility, but one couple stood out to me. The lady was in her late forties at the time, and her partner was in his late twenties. She was diagnosed with secondary infertility, and she was fine with the diagnosis taking her age into consideration. After several unsuccessful attempts with Clomid (a fertility drug therapy to promote ovulation), trigger shots, and timed intercourse, she was advised to look into IVF. Interestingly, it was only during the IVF process that her younger partner was diagnosed with male infertility, which sent a series of shockwaves through them.

It was so hard on him in particular because he didn't think a man his age with healthy lifestyle choices could be infertile. I watched him transmogrify from a very jovial guy to the complete opposite in no time. Anxiety, anger, frustration, and depression kicked in. He began losing his self-esteem and self-confidence rapidly. I saw him declining. Following male fertility treatment on him, they proceeded to do IFV, but unfortunately, that cycle resulted in a failure.

To say this young man hit rock bottom after his partner's beta test came out negative is an understatement. He blamed himself for the results and said he felt like "less of a man." He went into serious depression, and I saw less of him as the days went buy. He kept himself on a self-imposed lockdown.

The consequences of struggling with fertility in men are equally as severe as in women and should not be discounted. That said, let's look at some of the damaging consequences that are present among a great number of couples battling this colossal and hideous monster.

Medication Side Effects

Approximately 85 to 90 percent of fertility patients are treated with conventional methods that include drug therapy to promote ovulation, trigger shots to assist with the release of an egg, intrauterine insemination (IUI) to facilitate fertilization, drugs to prevent miscarriages, all the way to surgery to repair reproductive organs. There is also the more sophisticated and advanced assisted reproductive IVF technology, but only about 3 percent of fertility patients can afford it. In as much as such medical interventions offer help and hope to these couples, studies show that they may also bring additional stress, anxiety, and grief on top of what the patients are already experiencing from the diagnosis itself.

All these drugs and hormones come with a lot of psychological side effects. Many women I have spoken to who took synthetic estrogen clomiphene citrate (Clomid) to increase their chances of ovulation (including myself), report experiencing anxiety, sleep interruptions, mood swings and irritability, thinking problems, frustrations, and depression.

Relationship and Social Problems

Struggling with fertility influences a wide range of psychological, cognitive, and emotional processes in everyday life. It can contribute to a sense of identity and is often intertwined in a person's self-concept, which ends up taking a toll on his or her social life. It is not uncommon for relationships to suffer when a couple is struggling with fertility issues. Not only do primary relations with a spouse or partner suffer but also relationships with friends and family who may inadvertently cause pain to a couple dealing with this reality by offering well-intentioned but often misguided advice and opinions.

It is also common for couples to avoid social gatherings and interactions with pregnant friends and/or families who have children. They may also struggle with anxiety-related sexual dysfunctions for several reasons, one being that intercourse, which is meant to be a pleasurable thing that happens spontaneously elicited from sexual attraction, feelings, and arousal, all of a sudden becomes a scheduled job. It has to be done on a particular day and at a particular time irrespective of the couple's mood. This type of intercourse can lead to other marital conflicts and hurt relationships.

Although the majority of relationships tend to suffer during struggles with fertility, some couples actually get closer to each other. (I'm not by any means saying you need to be a fertility patient to get closer to your partner, by the way.) In my case, my relationship got even stronger during our struggle. This isn't because we breezed through the process without challenges. On the contrary, it's the struggle and the grief from losing our baby that prepared us for this challenge. It is the need for mutual support that brought us closer together and that led to a much stronger, more secure, and unbreakable bond between us.

Financial Problems

Although IVF is becoming increasingly popular among couples struggling with their fertility, the principal obstacle to parenthood for most couples is financial and not psychological when faced with these struggles. That said, let's take a deeper dive into IVF and finance.

Fertility treatment costs are significant, but unfortunately, most patients have to cover such costs out of pocket. In the United States, for example, only fifteen states are mandated to provide insurance coverage for fertility treatments but only to an extent. On average, it costs about $12,000 for an IVF cycle using fresh embryos, excluding medications, which usually run another $3,000 to $5,000. It gets even more expensive and complicated if a couple requires donor eggs and/or surrogacy.

The price tag may not present a problem to celebrity couples and couples with deep pockets, but the reality is that not very many people struggling with fertility are fortunate enough to fall in a high tax bracket. Couples who do not have an insurance coverage or who can't afford the treatment out of pocket are often left feeling helpless, hopeless, and depressed. Even patients with insurance coverage often report that either copayments are often too high for them to afford or that their insurance coverage has a lot of limitations that end up requiring huge out-of-pocket expenses for treatment.

A lot of couples have gotten themselves into serious debt in the process of seeking fertility treatment. For most couples, the price tag attached to IVF places the procedure out of reach, and the spiraling costs associated with the fertility industry in general means that the benefits of assisted reproductive technologies are not equally available to all.

Taking my situation into consideration as an organic example, I had to travel abroad not because of my love for travel but to seek affordable treatment because the packages available at home were way too expensive for me. Simply put, I couldn't afford them. Every single couple from developed countries I met during my journey expressed that they had no choice but to travel abroad (like I did) because they just couldn't afford the packages at home. Ninety-five percent of these couples were from the United States; 3 percent were from Canada, the United Kingdom, and

Australia; and the other remaining 2 percent were from Asia, the Middle East, and Africa.

Let me draw your attention back to the excerpts above from various celebrities. If you read in between the lines as much as I do, you probably realized that their struggle was not limited by finance as is the case with most citizens who fall in the middle class or below. Their concerns, though equally valid and genuine, are far from financial worry. I am in no way saying they don't hurt because they've got the money to spend. I'm simply saying with the kind of money they have, they are able to afford multiple IVF cycles and surrogacies in order to realize their dreams of bringing home a baby or babies.

Celine Dion, for example, could easily afford six IVF cycles back-to-back because she has the money. People like Giuliana Rancic, Elizabeth Banks, Angela Bassett, Nicole Kidman, Sarah Jessica Parker, Kim Kardashian, Gabrielle Union, and a host of others with incredibly deep pockets could easily hire surrogates to carry their babies for them and bring home a living baby because they have the funds to do so. The truth is that most people (including myself) who are battling fertility can't afford multiple rounds of IVF, let alone surrogacy.

Celine Dion said, "I thought as long as my health permitted me and unless my doctor thought physically I couldn't do it, then, I would go on with the IVF until someone told me to stop." Wow! I really wish I could say that. In the same excerpt, she went ahead to say, "People stop because it's very expensive but I kept on going." Really? Celine Dion was obviously very much aware of the fact that IVF is a very expensive procedure when she said this, but unlike many others, she kept on going because, hey, she can afford it and money is not her problem anyway.

For the average American, this is not the case, unfortunately. They can barely afford one IVF cycle, and in most cases, their finances are completely wiped out after they are done with the process. Some even go into debt just to finance one IVF cycle. Not only are they struggling with an emotionally daunting issue, but they are also limited by the financial factor, which leaves them struggling to raise money to fund their dreams of having a baby. What a salty situation to be in!

In developing and underdeveloped countries, some people can't even afford a consultation fee, so they end up never having the opportunity to see a medical professional to get a diagnosis. They never get to know why they are not getting pregnant. They suffer in ignorance and silence for the rest of their lives. What saddens me about this is that, in most cases, their conditions could probably be easily diagnosed and treated. Some face things as easy as ovulation problems that can be diagnosed with a few blood tests and treated with ovulation induction medicines and timed intercourse. But because they never get to see a doctor, they are left untreated. In some areas, the proper equipment for diagnosis is not even available, and hence, there is no means to actually know why a couple is unable to conceive.

Granted, developed countries do not have the same problems as underdeveloped or developing countries, but at some point during my fertility journey, I started feeling like I was in a rural area in an underdeveloped country. Where am I going with this? In developed countries, we have the finest facilities, equipment, and medical personnel, but I couldn't really tap into them because the best comes at a cost, I guess. I can see a doctor and get a diagnosis, but I can't afford the treatment available for my situation. Why do they exist when we can't afford them? The bottom line is that I am left untreated because I can't afford treatment.

So how am I different from that woman in an underdeveloped country who can't afford a consultation fee to see a doctor to examine her? After all is said and done, that woman and I are still unable to get our health conditions properly evaluated, diagnosed, and treated by the best medical practitioners because—you guessed right—we can't afford it. I can't help but visualize a world with affordable fertility treatments where people's ability to have children when faced with fertility struggles is not limited to how deep their pockets are. I hope, pray, and long for this every single day.

Mental Health Challenges

Many studies and reports indicate that fertility patients may experience serious mental health problems on a transient basis as they deal with the emotional and physical roller coaster typical of fertility struggles and treatment. Case studies and reports using self-report measures indicate that fertility patients feel more distressed than other people.

According to the American Society for Reproductive Medicine, a structured diagnostic interview with a psychiatrist was carried out in Taiwan to examine 112 patients who were seeking assisted reproductive treatment. Comparing results with a separate study that had been carried out in patients seeking general medical care, higher levels of anxiety and depression were found in the women seeking fertility treatments than those found in the general population. Twenty-three percent of the study population (women seeking fertility treatments) was diagnosed with anxiety compared with 11 percent diagnosed in other patients. Seventeen percent of the study population was diagnosed with major depression compared with 6 percent in other patients.

Fertility treatment not only causes depression and anxiety in patients, but it can also exacerbate existing psychiatric conditions. Fertility patients with a history of depression are more susceptible to depression, anxiety, stress, and other psychiatric disorders during treatment than other women.

Some of you may or may not have been wondering or asking why I got emboldened from Prince Harry's revelation. He is not a woman, he hasn't suffered a placental abruption, and he is not battling fertility. That's correct. He may not have suffered identical tragedies and struggles as me, but his struggles and mine both lead to a common severe consequence: mental health issues, which he admitted he suffered. Mental health issues are very present in our societies, but unfortunately, these issues are not widely acknowledged. As earlier mentioned, the prince in his April 2017 podcast interview disclosed that he suffered depression, anxiety, and other psychiatric disorders after losing his mom unexpectedly.

Being someone who hasn't fully recovered from an unexpected death experience, I feared for myself and felt this strong urge to research about the consequences of unexpected death, and my findings were crippling for a moment before I regained some momentum. Unexpected death is associated with the development of depression and anxiety symptoms, substance abuse, and other psychiatric disorders, varying across different stages of life. These findings solidified Harry's candid admission and got me evaluating myself. Not only was I dealing with unexpected death, but I was battling infertility, both elements carrying unpleasant *mental health* consequences.

Unexpected death and fertility struggles are both very stressful life events associated with icy-cold consequences clustered around manic episodes, phobias, alcoholic disorders, substance abuse, post-traumatic stress disorder (PTSD), generalized anxiety disorders, and a heightened risk of prolonged depression and suffering across the life course of the affected individual. Faced with both severe elements, I felt like the world was closing up on me.

Although I wasn't diagnosed with mental health issues yet, I was at risk of being attacked by these multiple psychiatric disorders. It wasn't unusual for me to feel a lot of anger and to get depressed every now and then. Being calm wasn't really my forte anymore. I was gradually adopting hostile behaviors, and a lot of things were taking a downhill turn in my character. In that moment, I came to the realization that I had to work on myself or ignore everything and crash and burn eventually.

Since then, I've learned to continuously make a conscious effort to protect my mental health. While it hasn't been a walk through the park, the results have been nothing short of amazing. My baby hasn't come back from the death, and I'm still on the fertility struggle bus, but I can safely say that I am a better version of myself today than I was before the scales fell off my eyes and I was enlightened on mental health and its ramifications.

Depression, no matter how small it may appear, is not healthy and can challenge your sanity if left untreated. If you are susceptible to this demon, I encourage you to do all you can within your power to stop it in its tracks and prevent it from proliferating. After all, isn't prevention better than cure?

The Fear to Speak Up

My journey has been such an eye-opener. For a long time, I felt so uncomfortable sharing my diagnosis with people around me. In as much as I had this strong urge to open up about my struggles, there was that constant fear in me that I would be judged and shamed if I did, so I kept a stiff upper lip and walked around with a broad smile on my face while bleeding severely on the inside.

Society doesn't make it easier on people like me to open up about their fertility struggles. Interestingly, many people out there are living like this not because they want to but because they are afraid of being associated with a stigmatized topic. They can't talk about it freely unless they realize you are going through the same challenge as them. They are afraid of being called "that infertile girl," "that girl who can't get pregnant," or even "that girl who can't have children." They don't want to be called "that girl."

Did you know that people who are battling fertility really want to talk to someone? They need someone who will listen to them, understand them, and even be there for them if they can. They long to talk to someone who will not judge them—someone who will not take their story and run with it like a track star, spreading it everywhere they go. They need that safe place, so let us be intentional about being each other's safe place.

Every couple I met during my journey expressed fear about speaking up about their reality. They were so uncomfortable talking about what they were going through, and even when they did, I could see them struggling and holding back a lot of information. They would constantly look over their shoulders in the middle of a conversation for fear that someone might eavesdrop.

While receiving treatment abroad, I stayed at the same hotel with six other couples who were receiving treatment from the same reproductive endocrinologist. The funniest thing is that when I first asked them (on different occasions) what the purpose of their trip was, they said tourism. No one mentioned health. I told them the same story. We had the same lie to tell. Tourism is such a convincing tall tale to tell someone in such a situation. Unfortunately, that lie didn't last long, as we ended up running into each other in the waiting area at the doctor's office.

I didn't feel offended about the fact that they had lied to me because I had used that lie too on the same trip more than once. It was only then that we became close to each other and started opening up about our various situations and challenges. It was such a relief to finally have the opportunity to speak to someone openly and freely who could actually understand the profoundness of my pain. They gave me a very precious gift—a listening ear, encouragement, emotional support, and, above all, a safe place. In as much as a few family members knew about my struggles, I didn't disclose every detail to them because they worry too much about me. I kept the heavy stuff away from them.

Just like me, these couples and many others have had their struggles boxed up for years. Most of them told me that their friends and family didn't even know they were taking fertility treatments. One of them said, "I just can't discuss these kinds of things with them, you know. My name will be all over the place, and I don't want that for myself. I might tell them when this is over, and we've had our baby." This is definitely not the ideal way to live. No one should live life like this. We all should be able to express ourselves about our struggles without any fear whatsoever.

Prior to meeting my lovely friends, life was bizarre when it came to conversations surrounding fertility. Permit me to narrate this example here. I will meet a complete stranger at the airport while in transit and spill all the contents of my precious secret box because I haven't had the opportunity to simply air my feelings without being judged. Also, I will feel very safe doing so because I don't know this person I am talking to, and this person doesn't know me, and the chances of us ever running into each other in the future are extremely slim.

At the end of our conversation, I will realize I don't even know this person's name, but I don't feel the need to ask because why do I need it when I don't want the individual to remember ever having this conversation with me? I will then pick up my belongings and say, "Thank you so much for listening to me. It was very nice talking to you. Have a safe trip," and I walk away feeling so much better until I arrive at my final destination and spot my friend or family happily waiting to pick me up. As we drive home, I am able to chat to them about all but one thing—my fertility battle.

Isn't that pathetic? Think about it for a minute. I just told a complete stranger the story of my life, but I don't feel free having that same conversation with the people closest to me. Why? Why can't I feel free to speak to my friends and family? Why do I have to run to complete strangers with pertinent issues? Do you see what taboos can do? Do you see how damaging stigmatized topic can be?

I made a lot of friends during my journey, and together we encouraged and supported each other as much as we could. We spoke on the phone every day and messaged each other multiple times a day. But on a deeper thought, one thing was missing: We never really got to know each other like you would with family and friends. All our conversations circled around fertility and babies. Conversations such as how many shots you've taken so far, what medications you are on, how many eggs were retrieved from you, when your embryo transfer is, and so on. Sometimes that can be draining. Who wants to talk about issues with fertility all day long?

There were days when I didn't simply feel like talking about this baby-making journey, but it never happened because one or two of my lovely ladies would either call me to talk about it or message me. It's like old people, you know. All they talk about is the weather and illnesses. They can talk about how many hip replacements they've had and their doctor's appointments and pillboxes all day, every day. When something is your reality, you find yourself talking about it over and over again.

Do I fault them? No. Why not? Because I know how it feels to want to talk about these kinds of things, but you don't feel comfortable to talk to the people around you for fear of being judged, labeled, and shamed. In as much as I may not want to talk about fertility at that particular moment in time, I think about the emptiness these ladies feel and the listening ear they need, and instantly, I know the right thing to do is to drop everything and be there for them, and I do just that.

The friendship between us might not be a regular friendship, but I believe we were placed in each other's lives for a reason. I continue to be there for them, and they do the same for me. I feel safe with them, and they feel safe with me as well. That's my idea of women supporting women. Regardless of the circumstances, you try to be there for a sister when she needs you.

When I came back from doing IVF, I resumed my daily activities, which included going back to work. I just couldn't stay at home for two weeks waiting to find out my results. That would have driven me mad. I needed a distraction and work offered that ... sort of. The downside to being at work was that I struggled with my medications and injections. I didn't want anyone to see my pillbox and start asking questions. IVF medications can be scary. The amount of pills you consume on a daily basis is unbelievable.

My organizational skills came in very handy during this period. I had my pills and injections neatly packed in some opaque round but tiny containers with days, dates, and times written on them so that whenever I had to pop a pill, I will just sneak into my purse, pick up exactly what I needed, and dash to the break room without raising eyebrows. This worked out pretty well, and no one ever noticed I was on any kind of treatment, but I still would have loved the freedom to speak up about my struggles. All of this engineering and extra preparedness stemmed up from the fear to speak up.

I had my moments during this period. Some days I would get into work, do my job, take my medications and shots in between, and go through the day without any stress, but some days were absolutely horrendous. I remember this one particular day vividly when I was actually just coming back from the bathroom from taking my shot and feeling all kinds of emotions and, at the same time, actively trying my best to conceal them with a fake smile like I always did.

As I walked along, I bumped into a coworker who stopped to compliment my outfit. It made me feel so good, but then she ruined it by saying, "You need to stop looking sexy and make some babies." She said so laughing, and then walked away as she waved. My goodness, did that burn! Those words cut me so deep I almost lost my mind. To say I was livid the rest of that day is an understatement.

But when you think about it, she had no idea that I was battling for my fertility. She had no clue that I was going through IVF. She didn't even know I was struggling with intense emotions. Had she known my situation, I don't believe she would have said such a thing to me. If I had the courage to tell her what I was going through, she wouldn't have said that. She probably would have been more careful with her words toward me. This is just an example of many unintended insensitive things that I have had to hear from people as I continue to battle for my fertility. It could be better if this issue got destigmatized, making it possible for people to be able to speak up freely.

CHAPTER 5

Combined Lessons Learned from Both Struggles

Tragic circumstances present us with challenges we simply cannot prepare for or be prepared enough to handle. Such challenges cause unspeakable pain not only for those who are directly affected but also for their loved ones who see misfortune befall them and watch them as they struggle with it. At some point in our lives, we all go through intensively painful situations brought either by the loss of a loved one, the news of a terminal illness or illness in general, setbacks, disappointments, and so on.

The harsh truth is that pain is part of life. It is inevitable. In as much we all love not to have setbacks, heartaches, disappointments, and so on, life is not a flowery bed of roses. We will all experience pain, and when we do, we need to find ways to cope. When I experienced my pain, I learned a lot of lessons, but four fundamental ones stuck with me, and I would like to share them with you.

1. Do Not Feed Your Pain

Pain is inevitable when you go through certain circumstances, but however dark the clouds may seem, be comforted in the fact that there is always a silver lining. Instead of focusing on the pain, find the silver lining in that pain and redirect your focus. Do not waste your pain. It is very easy to get discouraged when things do not work out the way you hoped or planned for. I didn't plan to carry a pregnancy for eight and a half months and then lose my baby to a placental abruption, and I didn't plan to become a fertility patient.

Faced with these monstrous circumstances, I accepted it as my new reality and began operating from a victim's perspective without realizing that I was doing myself a great disservice. I began losing interest in the things I enjoyed. Work was no longer interesting, and my dreams were no longer valid. I began feeling invaluable, started compromising a lot, and became very short sighted with no zeal to be excited about the future.

Slowly but surely, I became good at feeling sorry for myself and feeding myself with shame, guilt, mediocrity, and negativity. And what's interesting is that by doing so, I was equally attracting people who were feeding me with more negativity and causing me to compromise even more than I was already doing. It is true that what you feed will grow and what you starve will struggle and eventually die. If you feed your pain like I was doing, it will grow, and slowly but surely, it will destroy you.

When you are going through a painful situation, do not focus on the pain. It's already intensely painful to be in that situation. Why continue to feed it? What you should be doing is starving that pain and focusing on your dreams. Feed your values, your hopes, your dreams, your confidence, and your destiny. Do not dwell on thoughts of shame, guilt, fear, worry, and mediocrity. Do not give them any space in your mind.

Whatever has happened to you is in the past. It is history! Quit putting energy into negative events of the past. If you use your energy to feed negative events from your past, you will barely have any energy left to feed your dreams and fulfill your destiny. The only way you can let go of negative events of your past is to deliberately cause them to starve. If you do so, eventually that pain will get smaller and smaller, and before you know it, it will wither off and die.

I'm not saying you should become a superhuman with no feelings or emotions. I'm not saying you should never have a down moment either. We are humans with blood flowing through our veins. We have emotions and feelings, and when we've been struck by tragedy, down moments will creep in every now and then. I understand that fully well. What I'm saying is that you can't afford to let a painful event hurt you for the rest of your time here on earth. You can't let a season of mourning turn into a lifetime of mourning. At some point in your pain, you have to be bold, strong, and courageous enough to look at your past negative events right in the eye and say, "You are history."

It is not a very easy thing to do, but once you do it, you will feel so much better. Whatever it is that's causing you to hurt and keeping you in a black hole, let it go. You were not destined to be stuck in a black hole. You are destined for greater things—things that are far greater than you will ever imagine. Get up, dust yourself off, wear a smile on your face, put your passion and dreams back on, and move forward.

2. Turn Your Pain into Gain

When we go through pain, we hardly come out the same way we were before. Pain changes us. Interestingly, how pain changes or affects you as an individual is entirely up to you. You can come out better, or you can come out bitter. Some people come out stronger, more determined, and more confident with a new drive for success or with a new passion. They grow through the pain. On the other hand, some people come out completely shattered, disappointed, and defeated with no motivation to feed their dreams or pursue anything in life. They go through the pain without growing through it. They give up—just like I did initially.

We may never understand why bad things happen to us, but what I want you to know is that there is a purpose or a lesson in your pain. Instead of just going through pain, try and grow through it. If you go through pain without growing through it, you are doing yourself a great disservice. I know how uncomfortable and overwhelming it can be when faced with tragic circumstances. No matter how hard it may be, always remind yourself that there is a purpose in your pain and focus on that purpose. Have the right perspective. Adopt the attitude of a warrior and not that of a whiner. Don't let your pain break you. Put your foot down and get something out of it. Turn your pain into gain.

As weird as it may sound, once you go through pain, you are uniquely qualified to help someone struggling with the same or a similar situation. Today, I comfortably encourage people who are facing similar situations. I wouldn't have been able to do this had I not lived it and grown through it. I remember meeting this young, jovial nurse during one of my fertility treatment sessions. I knew nothing about her private life, and all she knew about me was the fact that I had fertility issues. One day she walked into the room to administer my injection with a frown on her face. Something seemed odd about her that day. I asked her what was going on, and she quickly dismissed it with a response of, "I'm fine." I knew she wasn't fine, but I didn't insist.

As she was about to inject me in the stomach area, she noticed a huge scar and asked me if I'd had a C-section before, to which I responded, "Yes, I have."

"Oh wow! I didn't know you had kids! How old are they?" she asked.

"Emmmm, I don't have kids yet. My baby didn't stay. He passed on," I replied.

She wanted to know more, so I shared my tragedy and my struggle with her, and she burst into tears, gave me a big hug, and told me I had no idea how much healing she had just gotten from my story. She said with what I've been through and all that I continue to go through, she is amazed that I walk around with such a beautiful smile on my face. She went on and shared with me the reason for the frown on her face.

She had suffered a miscarriage a few days earlier at five weeks of pregnancy, which left her distraught and disappointed. Comparing her situation to mine, she felt guilty for crying. She began expressing gratitude instantly, thanking me for helping her heal and acclaiming me for being such a strong woman. Seeing how much my story turned this young nurse's sadness around, I realized that no matter how hurt I may be about my circumstances, there is a purpose in my pain. The joy I experienced seeing a smile on this young nurse's face is inexplicable.

Although I didn't like my pain, I learned a lot from it. It actually built some things in me that would never have developed if I hadn't been through that excruciating pain. Believe me when I say that some things can only be developed in tough times. Today, I am stronger, more compassionate, more educated, more levelheaded, more confident, and so on than I was before my tragedy hit me.

If we could all use our pain for a cause, helping people who are struggling with the things we've already overcome, this world would be a better place. I believe you can find purpose in your pain and turn your tragedy into a positive. Let your test become your testimony. Do not waste your pain. Get your mind off of your pain and get out there and encourage somebody. In the process of doing so, not only will you stop feeding your pain, but you will start feeding a purpose, and that's when you truly begin to experience your own healing. Don't get discouraged when it's painful, for there is a purpose in your pain. Starve that pain and focus on the purpose, and you will find your healing.

3. Choose Your Worry

Worry causes us to either feel anxious, distressed, troubled, or uneasy. It may not be a very pleasant feeling, but it is actually a quite essential, normal, and instinctive emotion that has been hardwired into us as humans in order to help us survive since we rose out of the primordial muck. Worry is a normal part of life, and everyone does it. In normal circumstances when you worry about something, you take the necessary steps to protect yourself from any harm that could potentially evolve from the anticipated situation.

For example, when you worry about your financial future, you try to put plans in place to protect it. When you worry about an upcoming competition or exam, you intensify your preparations toward it. When you worry about your children, you do everything to protect them. Do you get the picture? Basically, when we perceive something as a threat to our existence, we worry about it and tend to focus on it in order to protect ourselves from the consequences that particular threat might pose to us. This kind of worry is called healthy worry. It is adaptive, and it is a completely normal part of life.

Worry, although a natural part of the human condition, can sometimes be unhealthy worry. When worry becomes too frequent, too intense, and too unrelenting, it can cut down on your happiness and enjoyment of life. That's the kind of worry I am concerned about. It is maladaptive and fuels negative and obsessive thoughts, doubt, physical anxiety, and fear. It makes you unhappy and puts you in a position where you find it difficult to enjoy yourself. Unhealthy worry also stirs up a feeling of fear in you and makes you unwilling to take reasonable risks. It even interferes with your regular activities.

Prior to my tragedy and subsequent fertility struggles, my worries fell into the healthy category: I worried about securing a stable career for myself, I worried about my financial future, I worried about being able to provide for and take care of my parents when they become fragile, and so on. This kind of worry pushed me to work harder in order to secure the kind of future I envisioned for myself. I was in control, and life was good.

On the other hand, when tragedy hit me, things changed to the negative direction. I began indulging in unhealthy worry, and life became miserable. I had lost control. I was so unhappy and found it difficult to have a good time. Unhealthy worry is maladaptive and can damage you in ways you've never thought possible. When I regained control and started focusing my energy on healthy worry, my life began getting better. I started enjoying the things I loved to do, and life in general became more pleasurable and worth living. Try your best not to entertain unhealthy worry. Identify it and stay away from it as much as you can. It is a very toxic thing to entertain.

4. Dealing with Insensitive People and Comments

Some people can be very insensitive, and I'm sure we can all attest to that. The truth is, I let that get the better of me in the beginning, but I'm proud to say that I've learned not to dwell on negatives anymore. I don't give it an audience. It's just not worth my time. As a matter of fact, I don't really fault anyone for any negative thing they've said or done to me regarding the circumstances I've faced and the residue I'm still dealing with. You know, everyone's view of an object is influenced by where they are sitting at a particular point in time.

Permit me to get my point across by using this simple analogy. Imagine someone asked a group of people to write an essay based on the view of a centerpiece from where they were sitting. The one limitation is that no one is allowed to switch seats to appreciate the view from another angle. The end products would not be identical. Why? Because each person would pen his or her essay based on what is seen, and what is seen is influenced by where the person sat.

So, it is perfectly OK for me to miss including very important features about this centerpiece that are located on the side that I can't see, and the same applies to you. At least we are lucky to be close to the centerpiece.

How about those who are sitting far away from it? Can you imagine what their essays will sound like when you take a read? You see why I don't fault people? I don't know where they are sitting. Instead of faulting people, I try to inspire, educate, and create awareness on these important things because knowledge is power. Going back to our centerpiece analogy, if these same people could have the opportunity to come closer to it and hold and take a better look at it, their essays would be different.

CHAPTER 6

Life and Its Events

In this life in general, we all must have encountered both positive and negative events at some point. If you sit back and think deeply, you will realize that we tend to remember the negative events far better than the positive ones. Even when we remember those negative events, we hardly try to find a silver lining in them. Why? Because it is human nature, so don't blame yourself. Science teaches us that the brain's amygdala is responsible for declarative memory or facts that can be recalled. The more emotionally charged an event is, the more amygdala is activated in the brain. That is why we remember negative events more than we do positive ones. Our brains are hardwired to react more to negative events, and as such, we must constantly make a conscious effort to train our brains to work in our favor. Have you ever pondered about any of the following situations by any chance? I have, and if you haven't, I urge you to do so.

1. Why do negative events cause us to self-evaluate and search for meaning?
2. Why are we more likely to remember an individual's negative traits more than the positive ones?
3. Why do our brains devote more time and attention to negative stimulus and less time and attention to positive ones?
4. Why do people tend to remember the negative word choices we use to describe them much more so than any positive attributes we list?
5. Why does rejection from our peers affect our self-esteem much more than acceptance?

Each of the above scenarios can increase the impact negativity has on us. We have to be aware of this in order to make the effort to stop our brains from focusing on the negatives and getting the better of us. We can train our minds to work in our favor. We can choose to dwell more on the positive events than the negative ones. If you don't control your mind, your mind will control you. Granted, you can't control the outside world, but trust me on this one—if there is one thing about you that you can control, it is your mind. Yes! You can control your mind. You are the CEO of your mind. Train it and shape it the way you want it to function, and it will succumb.

CHAPTER 7

Supposition

In all honesty, my adversities, troubles, obstacles, and struggles have strengthened me in ways I never deemed possible. I didn't realize when it was happening because I was too busy focusing on the problems and the negatives and not looking on the bright side of things. Although adversity can be gut-wrenching and can shake you in ways you've never imagined, it can also make you stronger and tougher. My struggles revealed a whole new side of myself to me and solidified the fact that however dark the clouds may be, there is always a silver lining. We just need to stay focused and keep looking till we find it. I strongly believe that sometimes it takes an overwhelming breakdown to attain an unfathomable breakthrough, so hang in there.

I also completely understand that this message might take a while to sink in for some people, but that is perfectly okay. Remember that when you listen to some songs for the first time, you might not completely relate to them. The tendency to say you don't like a song after the first listen is very likely. But if you keep turning on the radio and hearing that same song over and over, before long, you start getting familiar with it. Then, the next time you go partying and the DJ plays that song, you find yourself screaming, "That's my song."

My fervent wish is that—just like that song that takes a while for you to take a liking to—this message should slowly but surely make its way to the top of the list of the kind of messages you want to hear and associate with. That's the kind of strong finish I'm hoping for, and I strongly believe that we will get there.

To those who instantly relate and welcome this message, please chime in. Let's continue to clamor and educate on this topic as much as we can, and hopefully, just like that music some people didn't like in the beginning, they might one day say, "That's the message." I strongly believe that together we can do this and shift the norms. Thank you! Thank you! Thank you!